CHASING *LIFE*

CHASING *LIFE*

New Discoveries in the Search for Immortality to Help You Age Less Today

SANJAY GUPTA, MD

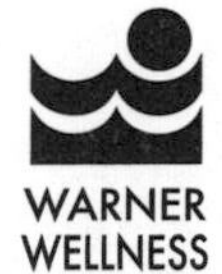

NEW YORK   BOSTON

This book is not intended to be a substitute for medical advice from a physician. The reader should regularly consult a physician in all matters relating to his or her health, and particularly in respect to any symptoms that may require diagnosis or medical attention.

Warner Wellness
Hachette Book Group USA
237 Park Avenue
New York, NY 10169

Visit our Web site at www.HachetteBookGroupUSA.com.

Warner Wellness is an imprint of Warner Books, Inc.

Printed in the United States of America

First Edition: April 2007
10 9 8 7 6 5 4 3 2 1

Library of Congress Cataloging-in-Publication Data
Gupta, Sanjay.
Chasing life : new discoveries in the search for immortality to help you age less today / Sanjay Gupta.—1st ed.
p. cm.
Includes index.
ISBN-13: 978-0-446-52650-0
ISBN-10: 0-446-52650-9
1. Longevity—Popular works. 2. Aging—Prevention—Popular works.
I. Title.
RA776.75.G87 2007
613.2—dc22 2006036951

Book design by Charles Sutherland

To my wife, Rebecca, and my daughter, Sage. Thanks for giving me the time to write this book. Please know that I thought about you both while writing every single word. And to my parents, Damyanti and Subhash, and my brother, Suneel, I hope we all achieve our own immortality.

CONTENTS

ACKNOWLEDGMENTS ix

CHAPTER 1 *BEGINNING THE CHASE* 1

CHAPTER 2 *LIVING TO A HUNDRED* 17

CHAPTER 3 *THE SUPPLEMENT BOOM* 47

CHAPTER 4 *RUN FOR YOUR LIFE* 75

CHAPTER 5 *MEMORIES R US* 93

CHAPTER 6 *TAMING THE BEAST* 119

CHAPTER 7 *A GROWING PROBLEM* 151

CHAPTER 8 *SUNNY-SIDE UP* 179

CHAPTER 9 *THE FUTURE IS COMING* 203

CHAPTER 10 *CHASING LIFE* 235

RESOURCES 239

READING LIST 249

INDEX 251

ABOUT THE AUTHOR 259

ACKNOWLEDGMENTS

David Martin is a good friend, thorough researcher, and fantastic writer. Without his help, this book simply could not have been finished. Like me, he is passionate about extending the lives of people all around the world. We stumbled upon the fantastic stories of stem cells for the rich and famous in Moscow and spent time learning from the wisdom of centenarians in upstate New York. David will also be the producer of the upcoming television documentary, also called *Chasing Life*.

CHASING *LIFE*

CHAPTER 1

Beginning the Chase

As I started to talk about my modern-day quest for immortality with colleagues and contacts I had developed over the years, I heard murmurs about a group of Russians who were convinced they had stumbled on the fountain of youth. More specifically, they were confident they had developed ways to achieve a sort of practical immortality. In fact, the word echoing through the longevity chambers was that we were rapidly arriving at a time when the only limit on life span might simply be an individual's decision to stop living. Visions of youthful 120-year-olds with several genetically perfect transplanted body parts, exchanged like a muffler or transmission, danced through my head. These Russians heard of my chase for life and started trying to make contact with me. Surely they wanted me to use my platform as a journalist to shine a light on their own work. Honestly, at first, I was skeptical, and it hardly seemed worth pursuing. As I read more and more about these doctors and the patients who stood to benefit, however, I became fascinated, if not obsessed.

Doctors there invited me to see firsthand what they called not only the slowing of aging, but the actual *reversing* of it. I couldn't resist, and with an Indiana Jones sense of adventure, I immediately took them up on their offer, which meant taking a trip to Russia in the heart of winter. As I disembarked the plane into the 20-degree weather, I mused to myself, "Okay, I get it, antiaging equals a deep freeze in Siberia." Still, donning a thick, gray wool scarf and one of those ridiculous hats with the earflaps, I started my chase for life.

It is in an upscale business district not far from the Kremlin that I meet Dr. Alexander Tepliashin. He is famous here because he offers something hardly anyone will turn down. With a smile and a series of simple injections under the skin, Tepliashin offers "youth" in just about ten minutes. Tepliashin euphemistically calls these injections "treatments" at his Beauty Plaza Health & Spa. He promises to not only make clients look younger but to revitalize their hair and skin and give them more energy. Not surprisingly, there is one small catch. What he is offering is untested and illegal in much of the world.

Tepliashin is a fleshy man with thinning hair combed straight back and a taste for Ukranian Captain Black cigars. His ultramodern clinic takes up the top two floors of a building on a street populated with such luxury shops as Versace and Cartier. An angled glass ceiling brings in lots of natural light, casting a futuristic glow on the furniture. A metal spiral staircase in the center of the lobby leads to treatment rooms on the second floor.

When I come in from the January air outside, Tepliashin greets me warmly and invites me into his office, where coffee and tea are offered all around. Through his translator, he tells me how he is a man of science helping people with a treatment that is in extremely high demand. He shows me articles he has written and informs me of his growing reputation across Europe. Still, there is something unnerving about him. Perhaps it is that he seems comfortable staring at me for several long seconds while not saying a word. Or could be the two all black clad Russian strongmen who are sitting rigidly near the back of his office.

From his desk, Tepliashin likes to watch his computer screen, which offers voyeuristic, closed-circuit views of the operating room, lobby, and elsewhere in the clinic. Small, red rectangles on the screen track any movement, such as a new patient walking through the front door or a young scientist rushing down the hall with small, red-capped vials. Tepliashin's gaze, even while talking, appears nearly constantly drawn to the screen, which gives him the air of a scientist in a Bond movie. Lab technicians, all of them attractive young women in tight, white uniforms, add to the *Dr. No* feel of the place.

Tepliashin stares at me firmly and proclaims that his treatments are safe without me even asking the question. More than that, he says with a nearly dismissive wave of his hand, he can guarantee results. He is so sure of his treatments, he has even injected himself, he tells me while rolling up his sleeves. It has given him a more youthful visage and lowered his cholesterol in the process, all from a treatment that took less time than a blood pressure reading. He strokes his face and runs his fingers through his hair. Other benefits, he tells me, include darker hair, more youthful skin, and more energy. Having never met him before, it is hard for me to tell how much Tepliashin has benefited from his own treatments, but I doubt he could look any more content than he did at that moment. Yes, his just might be the face of a man who has found something that has eluded adventurers for the last thousand years.

As I peer into a vial Tepliashin is shaking back and forth, he whispers two words loud enough for everyone in the room to hear—stem cells. Yes, Tepliashin is selling stem cell treatments right under the nose of authorities, who have outlawed them outright. In fact, he runs the best-known Moscow stem cell clinic, which even advertises on the Internet and boasts a clientele from Croatia to as far away as Paris. Coming from the United States, the scientific capital of the world, I feel woefully behind. In the United States, we still only talk about the *possibility* of stem cell treatments. Here in Russia, where abortions outnumber live births two to one, fetuses and their stem cells are in abundant supply, and they are being used at an ever-quickening pace.

Stem cell treatments have become part of Moscow's gossip mill and underground society. Rumors circulate about which well-known Muscovites have undergone them. The pharmaceutical billionaire Vladimir Bryntsalov boasted to the press that his once-pocked skin is now smooth as a baby's, thanks to stem cell injections. When the Ukranian leader Viktor Yushchenko's smooth complexion suddenly became discolored and pocked during his 2004 run for president, the common rumor among Muscovites was that stem cell injections gone bad were the cause. We later learned it was dioxin poisoning making him ill and riddling his face with the acnelike scars.

As I traveled through Moscow and visited various laboratories and "beauty clinics," I realized that many prominent Russian citizens truly believe they have discovered something astounding, so much so that watchdog organizations overseeing the clinics are willing to turn their eyes the other way when it comes to enforcing the law. Despite the widespread knowledge of their existence, cosmetic stem cell treatments are officially illegal in Russia. You wouldn't know it from the Internet, though, where you can find Russian-language sites offering the treatments. Some stories have reported as many as fifty stem cell clinics in the Russian capital. Not surprisingly, most proprietors at these clinics prefer to remain in the shadows and didn't want to talk. That was not the case with Tepliashin.

When we meet, Tepliashin proudly shows me around his clinics and describes the process: After a battery of tests, patients undergo an operation under local anesthetic during which he removes 5 grams or more of fat tissue from the abdominal area or the thigh. Technicians place the fat cells in a vial, where they are put in a solution and spun in a centrifuge. From there, the precious stem cells are extracted and placed in a special growth medium, where they are incubated. It turns out stem cells are located in many different areas of the body, including your bone marrow and even your fat. Once the cells have multiplied sufficiently, vials of stem cells are placed in a tank of liquid nitrogen to induce a state of hibernation, awaiting injection under the skin. This turns out to be a critically important point: because people receiving the treatments get injections of their own cells, there is no risk of rejection the way there would be with cells taken from fetuses.

Tepliashin says his clients get their money's worth. More than looking younger, Tepliashin says stem cell treatments make people live longer, too, reversing the effects of stress, bad food, radiation from X-rays, and viruses. In short, these treatments help people chase life. Imagine a lifetime of eating cheeseburgers and absorbing sunshine on the beach without sunblock potentially reversed, according to Tepliashin, by using your own stem cells to simply rebuild and rejuvenate your damaged cells with fresh, new ones.

It is certainly true that stem cell treatments have not undergone any of the sorts of clinical trials required in the United States and Europe that would confirm they are safe and demonstrate they are effective. Still, there appears to be no shortage of willing clients from Russia's moneyed elite and from elsewhere in Europe. Standing next to a squat, cylindrical vat of liquid nitrogen, a gloved technician lifts a tray holding as many as a thousand vials—representing about five hundred paying customers. The price tag is not cheap: €10,000 to €25,000 for a course of treatments ($12,000–$30,000). As far as I can tell, they aren't willing to wait for a *New England Journal of Medicine* article to tell them what they think they already know—that stem cells can not only stop them from getting older but can actually turn the clock the other way and make them biologically younger.

"They are used to a comfortable life," Tepliashin tells me. "They do not want to become old. They want to stay young. And we can say that it's a routine procedure. It can be done easily." Tepliashin is a sort of modern-day explorer in the quest for immortality, and he believes he has had the most success. Truth is, we won't know how much success for decades to come, but attempting to stop the clock of aging and stay young is nothing new. Over the centuries, scientists, alchemists, doctors, explorers, and others have tried to find or concoct rejuvenating potions or develop other ways to extend the human life span. Some of their would-be remedies for aging included items not likely to be found at a local health food store: dog testicles, a stag's heart, the breath of a virgin. History is filled with exotic elixirs offering the false promise of eternal youth.

Juan Ponce de León set out looking for the fountain of youth but wound up discovering Florida, by accident, in 1513. I can almost see the T-shirt. Ancient Hebrew and Hindu tales also told of bodies of water capable of conferring eternal life. More than two thousand years ago, Chinese emperors thought there was nothing more important than sending maritime expeditions in search of immortality. They weren't looking for life-giving water but the Isles of the Eastern Sea, where immortals were supposed to live. In ancient Greece, there was a belief that in a remote part of the world lived the Hyperboreans, a people free of all natural ills, with a life span of one thousand years.

In more recent times, scientists traveled to isolated regions of the Caucasus in what was the Soviet Union, chasing reports of extreme longevity. Soviet scientists claimed Russian citizens had lived for 145 years. The Karakoram Mountains of Pakistan and the northern Andes also gained a reputation as places where people were thought to be extremely long-lived. In all three cases, the tales of remarkable longevity turned out to be more about poor record keeping than magnificent health.

Despite all humankind's efforts, we have remained constrained by a life span that has an outer boundary set by the Frenchwoman Jeanne Calment, who died in 1997 at the age of 122 years, 164 days. Hers is the longest confirmed life span. Even the fittest among us get old. Jack La Lanne is still swimming into his nineties, but he has not escaped the aging process despite his lifelong devotion to exercise and healthy living.

In order to begin our collective chase for life, it is important to establish a few points before we get into some of the antiaging prescriptions. First of all, aging, in and of itself, is a major risk factor for ailments including heart disease, cancer, diabetes, Alzheimer's, Parkinson's, and a number of other conditions. Also, no one in the United States has officially died of old age since 1951, when state and federal agencies updated the standard list of contributing and underlying causes of death. "Old age" was dropped from the list that year. Despite this clerical fact, aging is a process that causes people to lose physiological function—from the cellular level to organs to systems—to the point at which they are vulnerable to heart disease, stroke, and cancer—the three leading causes of death in older Americans.

In many ways, it is much easier to describe aging than to define it. The symptoms of aging are both subtle and obvious. We don't see or hear as well, our hair turns gray, our skin wrinkles, our reflexes slow, our mind becomes less sharp, our muscles become weaker, our bones become more brittle, our lung capacity diminishes. These are the obvious signs of aging. Still, watching someone age is a lot like watching grass grow: if you look for changes every day, you will likely be disappointed. The aging process is a slow, ticking clock that makes each of us older next year.

Obviously, we don't all age at the same rate. Our clocks tick at different speeds. One person may be spry at eighty, while a second may be bedridden. Even in the same individual, change can occur at different speeds. Someone may be mentally sharp but suffer from heart disease. Another person may have weak eyes but healthy lungs. If we are lucky enough to make it to old age, we will certainly have a combination of strengths and weaknesses, compared to our peers.

One question we should ask—and I'll explore this in the book—is what keeps us from growing old even more quickly than we do. After all, we humans are relatively lucky. The longest-lived lion only makes it 30 years. Monkeys can live to 50 and eagles to 80. Only the turtle appears to have us beat on the longevity scale, with a maximum life span of about 150 years.

Not all creatures suffer the indignities of aging, though. Alligators, Galápagos tortoises, sharks, sturgeons, and lobsters keep on growing throughout their lives and show no obvious loss of function as they get older. The 50-year-old lobster will reportedly snap its claw closed just as quickly as a younger lobster.

Another important point: most of us would not choose to

live longer for its own sake. We do not want to extend our years if that extra time on the planet lacks a certain quality of life. We want to live longer, but we want a sound mind and at least a minimally functional body when we do. Given the choice, most of us would surely choose to live like an incandescent bulb—shining brightly until the moment the light goes out. We want to live longer and die shorter. It would be ideal if we could live the majority of our lives with the body of a young teenager. Consider this: if we were able to maintain our body as it is when we're eleven—when our healing capacity is at its maximum—we could live for an estimated 1,200 years.

Currently, most of us reach our physical peak between twenty and thirty and begin a steady decline after that. By seventy, we have lost 40 percent of our maximum breathing capacity, muscle and bone mass have declined, body fat has increased, and sight and hearing have gotten worse. We may want to chase life and live longer, but not at the expense of function, both of mind and body.

Truth is, when it comes to extending life, remarkable progress has been made in the last century. In 1900, life expectancy in the United States was 47.3 years, but that was an average dragged down by the huge infant mortality rate. The three leading causes of death in the United States at that time were pneumonia and influenza, tuberculosis, and diarrhea and enteritis.

In fact, when Franklin Delano Roosevelt signed the Social Security Act into law in 1935, workers were actually considered lucky to reach retirement age. The average life expectancy was

64 years when the federal government cut the first monthly Social Security check to Ida May Fuller of Ludlow, Vermont. Of course, if you were lucky enough to make it to 65, chances were you'd live another 12.7 years, having beaten some of the early killers—even back then. Ida May Fuller surprised everyone, including President Roosevelt. She lived to 100, while he only lived to the age of 63.

By the end of the twentieth century, U.S. life expectancy had risen to 76.9, and it continues to inch upward. At this writing, life expectancy for women in the United States is 80.4 years; for men, 75.2 years.

Public health measures such as ensuring clean drinking water and medical advances such as the discovery of antibiotics helped many more children survive into adulthood in the twentieth century. The challenge for science now is to help us survive and thrive in our golden years. The challenge is to help us chase life and also enjoy it.

Already, advances in medicine and public health have changed our concept of aging. Our expectations have grown. Technology has given us new faith in what is possible. Now, not only do we expect to make it to our seventies and beyond, but we want to remain physically and mentally active for years to come after that. We want our sixties and seventies to be a new beginning, not the beginning of the end. The good news is research has made tremendous advances, and there are many things we can do right now to improve the quality and length of our lives. And there are advances on the horizon that are more than promising.

Many researchers of aging prefer to consider what they call *health span*, not *life span*. They also use the term *active life expectancy*, meaning the number of years we can expect to live free of chronic functional impairments.

The goal of this book is to help you extend your active life. There is a lot of conflicting information out there, and I will distill it down for you and show the most effective choices you can make right now to improve your health and longevity. We all make choices every day that affect our lives. The sum of those decisions equals about 70 percent of the factors determining your life span. That fact alone should empower you to start making some changes that will increase your life span and your health span. Also, many choices you make as a young adult can have long-lasting consequences. Even at eighty, though, it is not too late to chase a longer, healthier life. I will shatter some myths along the way, and yes, I'll also talk about the cutting-edge science underway in labs around the world in such areas as stem cells, telomeres, nanotechnology, and more that may open the door to what some are already calling *practical immortality*. While I won't make you any false promises, you will be astounded at the small yet remarkably effective changes you can make today to put you on the path to chasing life. This book will explore where longevity research is heading and what you can do now—based on the latest research. How much can we do to alter our life expectancies? The short answer is plenty.

In the course of researching and writing this book, I've discovered some things that have already changed my own life. For example, eating well is important, no doubt, but eating *less* might actually buy you more years of life. All books will tell you to exercise, but it is the right types of activity, including upper body resistance training (no, not the StairMaster for sixty minutes every day) that will be of most benefit in the long run. Attitude makes a huge difference. Just the act of practicing optimism can help, as can spending valuable time every day decreasing your stress levels. I will show you how to do it reliably. Getting enough sleep at night and challenging your brain during the day in addition to socializing and maintaining hobbies all appear to be the keys to a longer, healthy life. I'll explain each of these keys to a longer life and the best ways to attain them.

Many books offering health advice focus on a single area. They may tell you how to keep your brain healthy or how to maintain peak fitness or how to lower your stress or how to sleep better. Some of these books are very good, but common sense tells us that we need a balanced approach between diet and lifestyle. In this book, I will try to offer that. I will also try to make this book a clear and concise guide that rises above the clutter.

Some of the advice may surprise you. For example, physical fitness can have a profound effect on your cognitive abilities later in life, and your mental outlook could have a profound effect on your long-term physical health. Taking lots of supplements, as many experts recommend, may not be effective whatsoever. Eating a low-calorie diet could trigger a cellular reaction that leads to a cascade of events ultimately leading to longer life. How much exercise and what kind you do can make a difference. Eating foods like dark chocolate and dishes containing the spice turmeric and drinking red wine, green tea, and even coffee can all help you live longer and healthier, with a dramatically sharper mind.

Many in the scientific community are thinking about ways to alter the human life span. They are imagining great leaps in understanding aging and dreaming up ways to counteract it. In their brave new world science, we will be able to replace worn organs the way you replace the worn brakes on a car; special enzymes or genetic therapies will rejuvenate our cells; microscopic nanobots will circulate through our bodies, warning of future health problems, which can then be addressed. Researchers are predicting stem cells will someday prevent such degenerative diseases as Alzheimer's and Parkinson's. These therapeutic advances could shatter what we now consider a human life span, extending it by decades or more. Ray Kurzweil, a futurist and inventor, thinks scientific progress is advancing so quickly, we will all be able to live forever—if we can only make it a few more decades.

Despite the flurry of activity in labs across the developed world, there is no magic elixir yet, leaving those of us who want to live longer, healthier lives to use the best information currently available as guideposts. Of course, there are no guarantees. People who live lives that are paradigms of clean living succumb to cancer, and others who spend years ignoring the best advice of doctors and others live into old age. After all, Jeanne Calment reportedly didn't give up smoking until the age of 117.

While there are no guarantees, we are not destined to a life span similar to that of our parents. Although genetics do appear to play a role in how long we live, studies suggest our DNA accounts for only about 30 percent of how long we live. The rest is up to us. There are some simple rules that we all know, even if we choose to forget them from time to time. Nothing else in this book will matter unless you make a pact with me that you will adopt the best health practices that exist today. What will we eat? How much will we eat? Where and how will we live? Will we smoke cigarettes? wear a seat belt? ride a motorcycle? Do we exercise? Lifestyle does make a difference. An astonishing 46.5 million Americans smoke, even though it will result in disability and premature death for half of them.

Nothing can stop aging, but we can take steps to increase our chances of living longer, healthier lives. For this book, I have looked at the burgeoning field of antiaging medicine. I will do my best to cut through the conflicting information out there and tell you what you can actually do right now and what treatments may be available in the future to help you age well.

We already know from closely studying our neighbors in other developed countries that lifestyle choices can result in living longer lives. More than twenty other developed nations, including Japan, the United Kingdom, France, and Sweden, have higher life expectancies than does the United States.

Many people in those countries have already learned that something strange happens as our bodies get older. While the process of aging does certainly continue, the incidence of age-related diseases starts to slow way down. The incidence of cancer, osteoporosis, and Alzheimer's disease becomes increasingly lower. It is almost as if our bodies and our minds realize that if they can get this far along, they could potentially go much longer and achieve a sort of immortality, which is the endgame of chasing life. My goal is to get you to the point where you are living longer, free of disease and of sound mind.

You won't need to inject yourself with illegal stem cells, and you won't need to travel to subzero Russia to achieve your own version of immortality—I have already done that for you. In fact, I have traveled all over the world to bring you stories of success, perseverance, and just good, old-fashioned clean living. Everywhere we go, we find one thing that binds us all together—we are all chasing life. Next stop: Okinawa, Japan, where we learn to live to one hundred.

CHAPTER 2

Living to a Hundred

Ushi Okushima has never missed a day of work at the bustling farmer's market in Okinawa. She can be counted on to have a bushel of the island's trademark small green oranges for sale. In addition to being a reliable presence, Okushima is very popular with the tourists, who often snap pictures and shake hands with the friendly fruit seller. Sometimes they ask to touch her snowy white hair. The reason Okushima creates such a stir among the island's visitors is her age. She is 103 years old. That is certainly remarkable by most standards, but not necessarily for the Okinawans. Residents of the 160 islands that comprise Okinawa are more likely to reach one hundred than people living anywhere else on the planet. Even in Japan, which boasts the longest average life span in the world, Okinawans stand out.

For starters, heart disease, stroke, and cancer occur at a lower frequency on Okinawa than anywhere in the world. Prostate cancer is unusual, and breast cancer is so rare, most women do not even require mammograms. You don't need advanced medical tests to see that many Okinawans, like Okushima, remain mentally and physically spry—and living independently—long past the age when devastating medical problems frequently trouble their counterparts in the United States and elsewhere around the world. On Okinawa, which lies between the main Japanese islands and Taiwan, there were 699 centenarians out of a population of 1.3 million in 2005, or 51 for every 100,000 people. Compare that to the United States, where there are only about 10 centenarians per 100,000 people.

It should come as no surprise that Okinawa has been a hotbed of aging research for decades. Scientists have drawn Okinawans' blood, taken their heart rates and blood pressure, scrutinized their diets and social interactions, interviewed them at length about their lives and their philosophy on life—all in an effort to learn what makes the islanders maintain such good health for so long. The question, of course, is whether they are genetically predestined to live longer, or whether there is something about the way they live that could benefit the rest of us. Simply put, can we live longer by becoming more like the Okinawans?

To answer the first question: Do Okinawans possess a "longevity gene?" The answer appears to be no. We know this for a simple reason. Okinawans who move away and adopt the lifestyle of their new country quickly develop life spans in line with their neighbors. That suggests their longevity results from the way Okinawans live and not to some genetic protection against the ravages of age. That means we should be able to learn a thing or two from them. So how do they live?

Well, this came as a surprise to me, but Okinawans do not enjoy an easy life. In fact, the word *retirement* does not even exist in the traditional Okinawan dialect. They work hard from an early age and don't stop working. In doing research for this book, I was told of a fisherman in Okinawa in his nineties who still dove from his boat every day for sea urchins. His family had begged him to stop, but he refused. As a compromise, he agreed to put his phone number on the side of his boat in case he dove from his small skiff and never returned. Asked about the secret to her longevity, Ushi Okushima talks about a strenuous life, not an easy one.

"We worked for long hours in the field," she says. "We grew and ate our own vegetables. We never spent our money on extra food. That's why I think I live so healthy." Okushima is by no means alone. Hard, purposeful work appears to be a theme among the centenarians in Okinawa. Fishermen, gardeners, and others continue laboring into their eighties, nineties, and beyond.

Okushima is often joined at the market by her seventy-six-year-old boyfriend. Her advice to others who want to duplicate her remarkable health and well-being: "Get a young man. The younger the better." I think she is joking, but given her success with longevity, I listen carefully to everything she says. This much is for sure: Okushima and other Okinawans not only work hard but have traditionally maintained active lifestyles throughout their lives. They grow up walking and gardening. Many also perform martial arts and traditional dance. So it appears more *activity*, not necessarily exercise but consistent movement, is associated with longevity, at least for the Okinawans.

The Okinawan diet, at least among the islands' elders, is little changed since the 1600s. It is rich in fruits and vegetables and unrefined carbohydrates. Staples include soups, soy products, and brown rice. They eat fish several times a week and consume minimal dairy products, fats, meat, or sugar. The traditional Okinawan diet averages about 500 fewer calories a day than the American diet. Although Okinawans are eating fewer calories, they are actually consuming a greater volume of food. That's because Okinawans' traditional foods are not dense with calories. The foods they eat contain a lot of water. The American diet is more energy dense. There is less water. The fats and sugars we like to eat contain more calories per gram of food. Burgers, pizza, and sandwiches—three of our favorite things—are all compact calorie bombs.

Possibly just as important, Okinawans have a tradition of pushing back from the table before they are full. This tradition is called *hara hachi bu*. I love this phrase and have been known to whisper it out loud when eating out with my wife. It means eat until only 80 percent full, and then stop. From a neuroscience perspective, this makes a lot of sense. That area of the brain that lets us know that we are really full usually lags several minutes behind our actual eating. So eating more slowly serves us well in terms of regulating the number of calories we consume. If you just wait a few minutes between bites, you will feel remarkably full, even if you were hungry just a few minutes before. Diet may not be the only key to Okinawans' long lives. They also share strong social ties.

Okinawans believe in helping neighbors, a practice of reciprocity called *yuimaru*. That may be one reason the Okinawans studied showed very low levels of stress. (I will look at stress, lifestyle, and outlook on life in chapter 8.)

Sadly, Okinawans' spectacular health may be fading as the western diet and lifestyle creep into their daily lives, thanks in good measure to the influence of a large U.S. military presence. Many younger Okinawans have adopted a taste for the pizza, burgers, and fried chicken available to the thousands of U.S. servicemen and women stationed there. In fact, Okinawans are now Japan's fattest people and have the dubious distinction of having the most hamburger restaurants per capita. In short, they are eating more like Americans. I think it's safe to predict that their prodigious longevity will start heading in the wrong direction, and their life spans will start moving toward that of their beefier friends living in North America.

EXTRA CALORIES ARE KILLING US

The eating habits in the United States remind me of the old joke about two people in line at a buffet. The first says, "This food is no good." The second adds, "Yes, and there's not enough of it." We are eating too much food, and the food we are eating is not good—at least nutritionally.

Let's consider how much we are eating. According to the latest figures available from the U.S. Department of Agriculture, daily food consumption increased 16 percent from 1970 to 2003, from 2,234 calories to 2,757 calories. That's an extra 523 calories per day. Fats and oils accounted for 216 of those additional calories. In fact, during those three decades, consumption of fats and oils increased an artery-clogging 63 percent, according to the USDA. It's no wonder we have bulked up as a society.

If you wanted to exercise off the excess calories we've added to our daily diets in the last thirty years, it would take some time. If you weigh 200 pounds, you'd have to walk for about 1 hour, 40 minutes to burn off those 523 calories. If you prefer jogging, it would take you 32 minutes at a 10-minute-per-mile pace. Remember, I'm not talking about all the calories consumed in a day. Not even a quarter. Just the *extra* 523 calories a day we've started eating, on average, since 1970. If you weigh 150 pounds, getting rid of those extra calories is an even more daunting proposition. You'd need to walk 2 hours, 13 minutes or jog 43 minutes at the same 10-minute-mile pace. These figures show clearly that it is much easier to eat less than to burn off through exercise what you've eaten. All those calories we eat but do not burn get stored as fat. There is an unforgiving math at work here. More calories in + same calories burned = more fat. This worked well when we were hunter-gatherers, but our evolutionary strategy for storing fat is a disaster now that food is so readily available in much of the world.

All the calories we're eating, combined with our sedentary lifestyle, have caused a spike in obesity rates in the United States. An estimated 65 percent of Americans—more than 175 million of us—are overweight or obese. Many other countries in the developed world have also seen a similar jump in obesity.

Worldwide, an estimated 1 billion people are overweight, and at least 300 million are obese.

On the Rise

The National Health and Nutrition Examination Surveys found that the percentage of U.S. adults who were overweight or obese increased from 55.9 percent in 1988 through 1994 to 65.2 percent in 1999 through 2002. Think about it. Almost two-thirds of Americans qualify as overweight or obese. Expanding waistlines have brought with them an increase in heart disease, diabetes, and other problems.

Dr. Barbara J. Rolls at The Pennsylvania State University is interested in the psychological and physiological controls of food intake. Basically, her goal is to figure out why we eat so much. For starters, she says, overeating has never been easier. At the same time, opportunities for exercise have decreased. Rolls and others in the field see growing portion size as a prime suspect. Exhibit A is the increasing number of meals we eat outside the home. There are any number of reasons for this, from busy schedules to growing commuting times to the increase in the number of families in which husband and wife both work outside the home. Eating restaurant meals generally means consuming more fat and saturated fat and less fiber and micronutrients than are found in home-cooked meals. Eating at fast food restaurants puts us in a position to "supersize it" and order meals that are not only inexpensive but gargantuan. Fast food is not the only place we can find hefty portions. As Rolls notes in a paper published in *Nutrition Today*, we can order muffins that weigh half a pound, 1-pound steaks, and bowls of pasta with 2 pounds of noodles. A "medium" popcorn at most movie theaters has 16 cups of popcorn—up to 1,000 calories. Even at home, Rolls says, portion sizes have grown larger.

Big portions mean bigger people, Rolls believes, at least in the United States, where we tend to eat what she refers to as energy-dense food. Remember, energy dense means a large number of calories for each gram of food. As I mentioned, the Okinawans consume a greater volume of food, but fruits and vegetables contain a lot of water and are not energy dense. Fruits and vegetables also contain a good deal more of the vitamins and nutrients we need.

Rolls does not think we need to throw our western diets out the window. Unfamiliar foods are generally less palatable, so advocating that people adopt an entirely new diet is a recipe for failure, she says. Instead, she says people should try to eat slightly smaller portions of the foods they like and make those portions slightly less dense with calories. That means less burger and more lettuce and tomato.

Rolls has written two books on the subject, offering readers the chance to experience what sounds too good to be true: lose weight while eating more. The cover of her book *The Volumetrics Weight-Control Plan* shows a quarter of a cheeseburger next to an enormous bowl of soup. There is an equal sign between them. The message: Choose food with a higher water content. That lets you increase the volume of what you eat while lowering the calories. You are eating more food and fewer calories at the same time.

If you could eat portions that were 25 percent smaller, and the food you ate was 25 percent less dense in calories, you'd eat 800 fewer calories a day, Rolls said. That is a huge number. Other researchers have suggested we could avoid obesity simply by eliminating 100 calories a day. If you eat an extra 10 calories a day—just 10 calories more than you burn off—you will gain a pound in a year. Keep that up, and by the time you're in your forties, you will have added 20 pounds to the weight you were on the day you graduated from college. Ten calories is nothing. A tablespoon of ketchup is more than 10 calories. Remember, Americans are eating 500 more calories a day compared to three decades ago. Of course, it is possible to go too far. There are some so obsessed with calories, they starve themselves to near death.

Rolls is also skeptical that we will be able to follow the Okinawans and push away from the table when we are only 80 percent full.

"How do people know they're 80 percent full?" she asks. "Most people don't know they're 140 percent full."

Again, it's not that our bodies don't send us signals telling us how full we are. They do. The signals come through both nerves and chemical messengers. Signals from the upper gastrointestinal tract are based on how distended our gut is and the amount of nutrients we've eaten. The signals are there. We are just very good at ignoring them.

Research has shown just how helpless we are at resisting the food in front of us. In one study, twenty-three normal and overweight people were recruited and fed over two 11-day periods, with a two-week break in between. During one of the 11-day periods, the test subjects received normal portions. During the next 11 days, they received portions that were 50 percent larger. This probably won't come as a surprise, but the participants ate more when they were offered more. On average, they consumed 16 percent more calories per day—4,500 extra calories during the 11 days. If they didn't exercise more, these test subjects would have put on more than a pound of fat in a week and a half—simply because they were offered larger portions.

Even when seconds are available, if you give diners a bigger portion initially, they will eat more. The way Rolls sees it, the only way to get people to eat less is to serve them less. In a society where many restaurants compete by offering ever-larger portions, this is not good news.

Researchers who have looked at people with severe amnesia offer us insights into just how poor the body is at alerting the brain we do not need more food—and just how vulnerable we are to overeating.

Probably the most famous amnesic in the medical literature is a man known simply as H.M. A surgeon removed a portion of the part of his brain called the frontal cortex, including most of his hippocampus, in 1953 to relieve his severe epileptic seizures. The surgery had the desired effect. It helped with the seizures, but there was one unexpected and profound side effect. H.M. was unable to form any new memories. This is known as anterograde amnesia. The hippocampus, a horseshoe-shaped structure in the brain, it turns out, is crucial for forming new memories. The past was intact, but H.M. lived in a perpetual present. Of course, the surgery changed H.M.'s life forever. He could not remember someone's face for more than a few minutes and would cry every time he heard his mother had died. He reportedly introduced himself to his doctor every morning. On one occasion, he ate a second complete dinner only minutes after eating the first one. Nothing in his brain registered that he was satiated.

The University of Pennsylvania psychologist Paul Rosin and his research colleagues decided to see how important memory was to appetite in an experiment with two other amnesics who, like H.M., could not retain new memories. They placed a meal in front of two men who could not remember anything new and announced, "Here's lunch." They reported what happened next in the journal *Psychological Science*: "Both patients (on three occasions each) readily consumed a second lunch when it was offered 10 to 30 min after completion of the first meal, and usually began to consume a third meal when it was offered 10 to 30 min after completion of the second meal." Their findings suggest that memory plays a big role in whether we think we are hungry or not. Looking at these results from a different perspective, our bodies appear to do a lousy job of telling our brains when we are full. Or maybe it's the other way around. Maybe our brains simply do a lousy job of listening.

Faced every day with a potential fast food smorgasbord, we appear unable to show the self-restraint of the Okinawan elders to push away from the table when we are only 80 percent full. Unlike the traditional Okinawans, we consume far too many calories and get few nutritional benefits as a result.

You've probably heard breakfast is the most important meal of the day. Eating a good breakfast may have more than simply nutritional benefits. Here's a tip that I now use just about every day. One way to eat fewer total calories during the day is to eat a bigger breakfast. Studies have shown that eating more calories earlier in the day appears to reduce the number of calories consumed overall. On the flip side, eating more calories later in the day is correlated with eating more calories overall. Calories consumed earlier in the day appear to satisfy our appetites better than those consumed later.

Of course, many Americans eat calories all day long. It's the national pastime called snacking, and Americans are doing more of it than ever. The average number of snacks per day is 1.6, up almost 50 percent since the 1970s. Not only that, the snacks we are eating contain more calories. Instead of succumbing to the temptations of the vending machine at work, bring some fruit from home and place it in a bowl in your cubicle or office. That way, when you feel like noshing, you can at least eat something nutritious. Too often, we don't.

THE ESSENTIALS

Even though we are downing more calories than ever before, we are falling short on some essentials that can help us be healthier and potentially live longer. According to a 2004 report:

- Half of us don't get enough fiber, vitamin A, vitamin C, or calcium in our diets.
- Two-thirds of us don't get enough magnesium.
- Nine in ten of us don't get enough vitamin E or potassium.

All of these are contained in foods readily available at the grocery store, and a shortage of any one of these can cause serious health problems in the long run.

Vitamin C

Let's look at what we can eat to do a better job of getting the right vitamins and nutrients in our diets, beginning with the most well known vitamin, vitamin C. With all the drinks that have added vitamin C, it's hard to believe 50 percent of Americans do not get enough of it. You don't have to drink fruit juice to get enough vitamin C; oranges and other citrus fruits, kiwi, raw red or green peppers, broccoli, strawberries, brussels sprouts, and cantaloupe are all good sources. Vitamin C is necessary for the production of collagen, the "glue" that binds skin, bones, tendons, ligaments, and blood vessels. Vitamin C is also necessary for the synthesis of a molecule that transports fat to the cells' power plants, called the mitochondria.

As an aside, cooking vegetables can take some of the nutrients out of them. For example, boiled vegetables can lose some of their vitamin C. Sometimes though, cooking makes the nutrients more digestible. That's the case with tomatoes. The lycopene in cooked tomatoes is more "bioavailable" than that from raw tomatoes. Fresh foods are generally more nutritious, but frozen foods can have more nutritional value than even fresh foods, because they are often picked when ripe and frozen right away. Canning requires heat, which can reduce the nutrients and occasionally involves adding unhealthy ingredients to improve taste. For example, canned fruits sometimes come in a heavy, sweet syrup, and salt is often added to canned vegetables.

An absence of vitamin C in the diet for a long period of time will result in scurvy, the dreaded and deadly disease that struck sailors on transoceanic voyages, with no access to fresh fruits and vegetables for months at a time.

The Scottish naval surgeon James Lind, aboard the H.M.S. *Salisbury* in 1747, figured out the connection between the lack of citrus fruit and scurvy in what many consider the first clinical trial in medicine. Lind took twelve men suffering from scurvy and divided them into six pairs. Each pair received a different potential cure in addition to their regular diets. There were cider; vinegar; seawater; sulfuric acid (given the pleasant-sounding name elixir of vitriol); a combination including garlic, mustard, and horseradish; and two oranges and one lemon daily. As we all know, those who ate the fruit experienced what Lind described as "the most sudden and visible good effects." Unfortunately, Lind's conclusive results were not widely accepted, and the Royal Navy did not require its sailors to have a daily ration of lemon or lime until 1795. When the dietary requirement went into effect, of course, it led to British sailors acquiring the nickname "limeys." Now we know that all that is needed to ward off scurvy is a spoonful a day of lemon or lime juice.

You don't have to be vitamin C-deprived to the point of

scurvy for the shortfall to cause health risks. Vitamin C is an antioxidant, and studies suggest it reduces the risk of heart disease, stroke, and cancer.

A single 8-ounce glass of orange juice meets the daily requirement. Somehow, half of us miss the mark on this vital vitamin.

Vitamin A

Vitamin A is often associated with vision. Vitamin A deficiency is the leading cause of blindness in the developing world. Sweet potatoes, carrots, spinach, kale, and winter squash all contain significant amounts of vitamin A, which is also required for a normally functioning immune system. Vitamin A may also lower the risk of macular degeneration, a deterioration of the central portion of the retina and the leading cause of blindness in those fifty-five and older in the United States. Eat a medium-sized sweet potato or a cup of either cooked carrots or cooked spinach, and you have achieved close to your daily requirement.

Vitamin E

Vitamin E is an antioxidant that appears to play a role in immunity and to have other benefits. Such nuts as almonds, peanuts, hazelnuts, and sunflower kernels contain significant amounts. Avocados and sunflower and safflower oils also contain vitamin E, as do olive oil, corn oil, and soybean oil, though in smaller amounts. They help protect the cell membranes from what are known as free radicals, which cause damaging oxidation in the body's cells. For example, the oxidation of proteins in the lens of the eye appears to cause cataracts, which may be prevented by taking antioxidants, such as vitamin E.

Severe vitamin E deficiency results in loss of balance and coordination, muscle weakness, and damage to the retina. Several large-scale studies suggest taking vitamin E may decrease the risk of heart attack and heart disease in men and women, although other studies have shown no such benefit. A Harvard study of more than 120,000 women and men found those with the most vitamin E in their diet were the least likely to get Parkinson's disease.

Many breakfast cereals are vitamin fortified and provide at least some of the vitamin E you need (that will be more easily absorbed by the body than vitamin E from a supplement). A little more than 2 ounces of almonds also gives you the daily requirement. Keep in mind, though, that nuts are packed with calories. For example, every ounce of almonds has 160 calories.

Vitamin D

Vitamin D is needed to maintain calcium levels in the body, which is essential for the normal functioning of the nervous system. Most of us need five or six times the amount of vitamin D we are getting.

We get some vitamin D when ultraviolet-B (UVB) light from sunlight activates a chemical in our skin. We also get vitamin D from fortified milk. According to the Harvard School of Public Health, if you live north of an imaginary line stretching from Philadelphia to San Francisco, where there is little sun for long stretches between October and March, chances are you are not getting enough vitamin D. Also, African Americans and others with dark skin, like me, in general have lower levels of vitamin D, because we do not produce as much of the vitamin.

As we get older, we become less efficient at converting the chemical in our skin to vitamin D. Also, many elderly people are careful about covering up and using plenty of sunscreen to protect against skin cancer. As a result, many seniors are not getting enough vitamin D. The result can be muscle pain and weakness. If you are older and fall into one of these categories, you should consider spending more time in the sun or taking a vitamin D supplement.

Fiber

Dietary fiber, the indigestible part of grains, fruits, and vegetables, promotes healthy bowel activity and helps keep our blood sugar in check. On average, we are only getting a little more than half the fiber we need in our diets. High-fiber cereals, whole-grain breads and such beans as lentils are good sources of fiber. The fiber they contain travels from the small intestine to the colon intact.

A number of studies have found that increasing the amount of fiber we eat from sources like legumes (beans, peas, and lentils) and food containing oats decreases our low-density lipoprotein (LDL), or "bad" cholesterol. Fiber-rich diets appear to lower the risk of heart disease and diabetes, although recent studies suggest it may not protect us from colorectal cancer, as we once believed.

Whenever possible, we should try to eat high-fiber foods, such as whole-grain bread, brown rice, fruits, and vegetables, instead of low-fiber foods, such as white rice, white bread, and chips.

While I'm on the topic of grains, I should mention that unprocessed foods tend to be more nutritious than processed foods. That's because processing removes nutrients and other beneficial elements from food. For example, whole grains have three layers: an outer layer rich in fiber, a starchy middle layer high in carbohydrates, and an inner layer rich in vitamins and minerals. Refining grain removes the outer and inner layers, leaving the starchy—and least nutritious—middle layer. Processing can also add trans fats, salt, and sugar, which may not be healthy.

Potassium

Let's consider some of the minerals we need, beginning with potassium. Fruits and vegetables contain potassium. The most potassium-rich fruits are dried prunes (and prune juice), raisins, bananas, oranges (and orange juice), and tomatoes (and tomato juice). A medium baked potato, with the skin, has more potassium than any of these. Other vegetables loaded with potassium are lima beans, artichokes, acorn squash, and spinach.

Potassium, along with sodium, is involved in creating an electrochemical charge across a cell membrane. This doesn't sound like much, but it is critical to a functioning heart, the transmission of nerve impulses, and muscle contractions. Prolonged vomiting or diarrhea can cause an excessive loss of potassium, which results in fatigue, muscle weakness, cramps, constipation, and abdominal pain.

Several large studies have linked an increase in potassium in the diet with lower blood pressure and a decreased risk of stroke, although the extent of the benefit and those who benefit differ from study to study. The potassium in fruits and vegetables also appears to help slow bone mineral density loss in elderly women and men.

Magnesium

Magnesium is found mostly in the skeleton, tissues, and organs. The mineral plays a role in more than three hundred essential metabolic reactions. It also helps keep bone strong and maintains nerve and muscle function, including the steady beating of our hearts. If you are eating a balanced diet, it's unlikely you will be dangerously magnesium deficient, because the kidney is able to limit how much of the mineral you excrete in your urine. But remember, two-thirds of us don't get enough magnesium. Because the same fruits and vegetables that have magnesium also have potassium and fiber, it is hard to state magnesium's benefits with certainty. There does appear to be some association between eating foods containing magnesium and lower blood pressure. Also, magnesium is associated with maintaining bone mineral density in elderly men and women.

Magnesium is present in chlorophyll, the green pigment in plants, so eating green, leafy vegetables is a good way to get magnesium in your diet. Bran cereal, oat bran, shredded wheat, brown rice, almonds, cashews, hazelnuts, peanuts, bananas, and milk are also good sources of magnesium.

Calcium

Calcium is the most common mineral in the body. Almost all of it is found in the bones and teeth. Calcium also plays a vital role in the blood, the fluid surrounding cells, nerve impulse transmission, muscle contraction, and hormone secretion. It is involved in blood clotting and the relaxation and constriction of blood vessels. Calcium is so important, the body will pull calcium from bones to keep blood calcium levels at the proper concentration. Not surprisingly, having a diet chronically low in calcium will result in less than ideal bone mass, quicker than average bone loss, and, eventually, osteoporosis. With osteoporosis, bone strength is diminished, and the risk of fracture goes up. Osteoporosis also poses a serious threat to long-term health. Nearly one-third of those who suffer a hip fracture as a result of osteoporosis enter a nursing home within a year. One in five people who suffer a hip fracture as a result of osteoporosis dies within a year. Sources of calcium are no secret: milk, yogurt, and cheese. Also, tofu, salmon, Chinese cabbage, and rhubarb contain significant amounts of calcium.

Iron and B Vitamins

Anemia is another serious problem among the elderly. One in eight elderly Americans—3.4 million Americans in all—suffers from anemia, meaning they do not have sufficient hemoglobin in their blood cells. I have met many elderly patients who complained they weren't feeling "right." They complained of general tiredness and loss of pep. Many times, it turned out to be anemia. Hemoglobin carries oxygen from the lungs to other tissues and returns carbon dioxide to the lungs. Someone who is anemic can feel tired, weak, dizzy, apathetic, and irritable. The most common causes of anemia are vitamin and mineral deficiencies, particularly iron, vitamin B_{12}, and folic acid. Changes in diet can help in some cases. Others require vitamin supplements or medication.

According to one study, anemia doubles the risk that an older person will develop serious physical problems that may jeopardize that person's ability to live independently. The study, sponsored by the National Institute on Aging and others, followed 1,146 people seventy-one and older for four years and measured their ability to perform a variety of physical tasks, such as balancing while standing and rising from a chair. Their scores on the physical tasks were compared with hemoglobin levels in their blood. Even those people whose iron levels were low but still above the traditional cutoff for anemia had 1.5 times the risk of developing serious physical decline. The solution might be as simple as taking iron sulfate pills.

MINIMIZE, NOT SUPERSIZE

Let's be honest. Maintaining a perfect diet or even a good one with our hectic lifestyles is extremely difficult. How many of us can honestly say we have not been in the drive-through lane at a fast food restaurant in the last month or two? But even if you are eating fast food on occasion, you can make choices that minimize the calories and fat you are consuming. For example, if you order the Quarter Pounder with Cheese, medium fries, and a medium Coke at McDonald's, you will consume 1,100 calories and 45 grams of fat (78 percent of the recommended daily intake). I've singled out McDonald's, but most fast food restaurants offer more or less the same choices.

Skip the fries, and drink water instead of a soft drink, and you've cut the calories by more than half and the fat by almost half. And the water is good for you. Believe it or not, despite the explosion of companies selling bottled water, many of us are not drinking enough water. Perhaps our love of soft drinks has caused this shortfall. I can't think of any other explanation. It goes without saying that water ranks right up there with air as an essential for living. Water helps maintain the body's temperature and transports nutrients. It also carries oxygen, keeps joints and organs functioning well, and washes away wastes and toxins.

What is it about fatty foods that make them so irresistible? The answer may be on the tip of our tongues, literally. Our tongues appear to be exquisitely sensitive to fat, which was a treasured foodstuff in hunter-gatherer times, but is now so abundant in our diets, we have trouble avoiding it.

Eating is without a doubt one of the great pleasures of life. As a neurosurgeon, I sometimes need to warn patients with frontal lobe tumors that the surgery to remove the tumor may damage the delicate nerve that connects the smell receptors in the nose to the brain. The nerve is exposed and hard to avoid when removing some tumors. Invariably, patients dismiss this potential consequence as no big deal. Only later, when they are confronted with a world without smell, do they express their dismay. Food no longer has the taste—or gives the pleasure—it once did, and this is a greater than expected sacrifice in quality of life. Deprived of the pleasure of eating, these smell-deprived individuals invariably lose weight, and they almost always tell me how the loss of most of their ability to taste has diminished their quality of life. I remember one young woman who required an operation in which I was forced to cut the olfactory nerves, those responsible for smell. At first, she didn't complain, but when I saw her back in my clinic a few months later, she had lost nearly 30 pounds. She described choosing foods more for consistency than for taste, which was nearly lost to her when she lost her smell. She no longer enjoyed pasta, which had been one of her favorite foods. To be sure, she liked the weight loss, but she missed her love affair with food. Most of us have the opposite problem; we are seduced by the aroma and taste of food, especially fatty food. But the next time you are feeling full and thinking about shoveling down another bite, remember the amnesic eating multiple meals. Or, better yet, repeat the Okinawan mantra: *hara hachi bu*.

EAT LESS, LIVE MORE?

There is a small group of dedicated individuals trying to one-up the Okinawans in order to extend their lives. These are adherents of a calorie-restricted diet. They eat enough to live, but nothing more. This is called undernutrition without malnutrition.

If pushing away from the table when we are 80 percent full is beneficial to our health, how about eating a lot less?

The scientific basis for this ascetic diet is based on research with rats. Since the 1930s, studies have shown that reducing the caloric intake of young or middle-aged lab rats by roughly a third—while maintaining their nutrition—increases their life span by 30 percent. They are also less susceptible to diseases, including diabetes and cancer.

This has prompted some people to cut their diets and their physiques to the bone. Their reasoning is simple: what works for rats in the lab will work for humans out in the world. What this group of diehards sacrifice in quality of life, they hope to get back in quantity. The motto of the Calorie Restriction Society? "Fewer calories. More life." Their belief is that calorie restriction is the only proven life-extension method known to modern science.

Researchers at Washington University in St. Louis have studied some adherents of the calorie-restricted diet. Not surprisingly, they were leaner and had lower blood pressure, more "good" cholesterol, less "bad" cholesterol, and fewer indicators of inflammation than the average American. These are all measures that suggest a lower risk of diabetes, heart attack, and stroke.

In 2006, the National Institute on Aging completed a comprehensive, first of its kind, six-month study of a calorie-restricted diet involving forty-eight slightly overweight but otherwise healthy men and women. They were divided into four groups. One group had their calories cut by a quarter. Another group combined a 12.5 percent calorie cut with a 12.5 percent increase in exercise. Members of a third group subsisted on an 890-calorie a day liquid diet for three months, or until they lost 15 percent of their weight, followed by weight management for the remaining three months. The fourth and final group, the control, simply aimed to keep their weight steady with a healthy diet containing less than 30 percent fat. The two groups that were not on the liquid diet ate a diet high in fruits and vegetables, with less than 30 percent of the calories coming from fat.

The results were striking. The average weight loss among those following the calorie-restricted diets was 18 pounds. More important, as far as the researchers were concerned, blood tests showed those who followed the low-calorie diets had significant decreases in the amount of age-related DNA damage, compared with their levels at the start of the test. Not only that, their metabolism slowed more than you would expect based on the amount of weight they lost. Also, their insulin levels and temperatures dropped. Along with the decrease in DNA damage, these last two factors may be the most important in terms of chasing life. Low fasting insulin level and body temperature are linked to longevity, according to the Baltimore Longitudinal Study of Aging, an ongoing, federally funded study that began in 1958.

The study couldn't say whether these people will live any longer as a result of cutting their calories, but the results certainly looked promising in terms of their health. This was the first phase of federally funded calorie-restriction research on humans. The goal was to ensure research on calorie restriction could be conducted safely and to see if researchers could recruit and retain test subjects. Only two of the forty-eight participants dropped out, and one of them was in the control group. Later in 2006, they planned to begin the second, two-year phase, with 240 people at three sites across the country.

With enough self-discipline, we are all able to choose a calorie-restricted diet. But for millions of years and in much of the animal kingdom, not getting enough food is not a choice but an unfortunate turn of events. Our ability to cope with fewer calories by slowing our metabolisms and making other changes in our metabolism worked well when we were hunter-gatherers and needed to endure lean times. Many other species have evolved ways to slow their metabolisms when food is scarce. Lower organisms are able to go into a sort of suspended animation. Mammals such as squirrels and bears hibernate. Most of us are fortunate enough not to endure any involuntary famines. It is a time of abundance, and calories are cheap.

"We are living in a constant feast. Our ancestors were living in periods of feast or famine," says Eric Ravussin, lead researcher on the calorie-restriction study, which was conducted at the Pennington Biomedical Research Center in Baton Rouge, Louisiana. "We need exercise just to get rid of the *extra* calories."

Life for the calorie restricted is not easy. Researchers in the field like to ask, "With caloric restriction, do you live longer, or does it just seem like it?" Even if a calorie-restricted diet is proven beyond any doubt to confer extra years on its adherents, would it be worth it? Those who follow the harsh diet appear gaunt, and their lower body temperature means they need to wear more clothes to avoid feeling cold. Researchers report other side effects, including loss of libido, low energy, irritability, and signs of depression. True believers counter that calorie restriction leads to inner harmony.

Another possible way to get the benefits of a calorie-restricted diet without the daily grind of eating the fewest calories possible to stay healthy may be regular fasting. Evidence from studies with laboratory animals suggests that eating every other day appears to offer the same enhanced longevity, even though the animals were consuming about the same number of total calories. Not only did the mice in studies manage to consume the same number of calories, but they didn't lose weight. Even so, intermittent fasting appears to offer the same or better results in some measures, such as lowering blood sugar. I'm not sure fasting every other day is a whole lot more palatable than following a calorie-restricted diet, but it, too, has attracted a good deal of interest from gerontologists and others.

How calorie restriction works to extend life is not known, but researchers have uncovered clues to some potential answers. Calorie restriction triggers genes that appear to promote cell survival, improve DNA stability, increase cellular repair mechanisms, and improve energy production and use. The lower body temperature and slower metabolism that result from calorie restriction may result in less genetic damage and lower the production of damaging free radicals.

The Hormesis Hypothesis

The beneficial results of calorie restriction may be a function of the hormesis hypothesis. The hormesis hypothesis says something bad in small doses can condition you to withstand something really bad in large doses. So a few minor, low-level stresses can activate stress-protective responses, so you are better prepared to withstand stress in general.

The ultimate answer may involve biological pathways not yet discovered. Needless to say, calorie restriction as a means to live longer is a topic of intense interest among those who have devoted their lives to figuring out the biology of aging. I don't think it's likely to become a widespread fad anytime soon, not when there are so many calories beckoning us everywhere we turn. As with so many other aspects of our lives, we are most likely going to look for an easier alternative, and there are several in the works.

EAT TO LIVE

So what should we eat to emulate the long-lived Okinawans? Remember, the traditional Okinawan diet is low in overall calories and rich in fruits, vegetables, fiber, and fish. The fish they eat contains omega-3 fats, which are thought to help protect the brain. Fiber helps the heart (more on this in chapter 7). Soybeans and colorful fruits and vegetables contain flavonoids, which are thought to promote health and ward off disease.

The U.S. Department of Agriculture (USDA) recommends five to nine servings of fruits and vegetables a day. The average Okinawan elder eats seven servings of fruits and vegetables a day. The traditional Okinawan diet also includes seven servings a day of grains, such as noodles and rice, plus green tea, fish, and soy foods, such as tofu.

To eat more like an Okinawan, look for deeply colored fruits and vegetables. They contain more flavonoids, vitamins, and antioxidants (more on antioxidants in chapter 3) than less colorful produce. For example, spinach, collards, and kale have more vitamins than iceberg lettuce, and sweet potatoes are more nutritious than white potatoes. Bright fruits include oranges, strawberries, and blueberries.

But don't stop there. The American Dietetic Association (ADA) launched the "Get a Taste for Nutrition" campaign to appeal to our more adventurous side, urging us to add a new fruit or vegetable to the shopping list each week. The ADA recommended we try kumquat, passion fruit, pomegranate, kohlrabi, bok choy, jicama, and parsnip.

Finally, we need to remember our Okinawan mantra: *hara hachi bu*. We need to push away from the table when we are only 80 percent full. Be aware of how much you have eaten, and remember that the brain appears to do a lousy job of listening to signals about how full we are. Forget that you can eat more. Forget how good the food is. Forget that your mother told you to eat everything on your plate. Just say *hara hachi bu*.

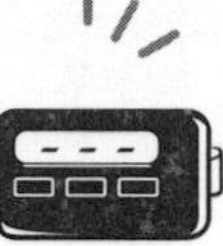

Paging Dr. Gupta

- ✓ Remember *hara hachi bu.*
- ✓ Eat only until you are 80 percent full.
- ✓ Find water-rich foods.
- ✓ Less burger and more lettuce.
- ✓ Slow down: Your brain needs a few minutes to signal you are full.
- ✓ Eat a bigger breakfast: You'll eat less the rest of the day.
- ✓ Eat less, and you may live more.
- ✓ Remember the essential vitamins you need every day.

CHAPTER 3

The Supplement Boom

As an information technology consultant with her own business, Laura Brown is used to tackling complex problems. Her specific field is computer architecture, and her clients have included Ernst & Young, General Electric, and Delta. She spends hours every day doing research before she makes any decisions. Her job depends on it. It is no surprise then that she approaches her health with the same degree of rigor. She is constantly searching for the best ways to maintain her well-being. After years of looking, Brown has come to her own simple conclusion: herbs and supplements are part of the formula for chasing life.

Brown has gone so far as to develop her own individualized plan for good health. In addition to vitamins, Brown takes three or four capsules of Chinese herbs twice a day. The fifty-two-year-old also drinks two or three cups of tea made from the passion flower daily as a way to help lower her blood pressure and ease the lower back pain that comes from spending long hours at the computer. She also occasionally takes a supplement made from the muscadine grape as an anti-inflammatory and antioxidant.

Brown, whose business is named System Innovations, also tries to keep her system finely tuned with aromatherapy. She attended a seminar in southern France to study aromatherapy several years ago and now uses such scents as lavender and peppermint for purposes ranging from relaxation to waking up.

Overall, Brown says her health is good, and she rarely needs to see a doctor. Since she began taking herbs and supplements, Brown says she no longer suffers from an annual cold. She is one of the 45 million who believe that taking natural products works to strengthen and support her natural defenses.

"Somewhere along the way I made a choice," says Brown, who speaks in a quiet way that belies her high-powered job. "I found an approach that worked."

Like Brown, millions of Americans are also choosing herbs and supplements, and the marketplace has responded with a myriad of purported remedies for all that ails us. Nowhere is the noise as loud as it is with antioxidants. Stories about antioxidants have graced the covers of national newsmagazines and the front pages of newspapers large and small. Food products claiming to be antioxidants are everywhere. Wander down almost any supermarket aisle, and you are likely to see products boasting their potential as antioxidants, from green tea to cereal to blueberries.

Just what does it mean to be an antioxidant?

ANTIOXIDANTS

More than thirty years ago, the Duke biochemistry graduate student Joe McCord was looking for the function of one obscure enzyme when he accidentally stumbled on another. He was so intrigued that he immediately called his mentor, Irwin Fridovich, to take a look. McCord had found a substance in the body that seemed to exist in every living species. As far as they could tell, this protein existed in the cells of all mammals, plants, and even microbes. Every single one of them. Right up the food chain. The only living organisms whose cells didn't have the enzyme were anaerobic bacteria—bacteria that do not need oxygen to survive. Initially, McCord and Fridovich didn't know what this enzyme did, but they knew it must be important. After all, every oxygen-breathing creature had selected for this enzyme during millions of years of evolution. The two researchers had discovered a protein, which they named superoxide dismutase, or SOD, that neutralized superoxide, an unstable and dangerous oxygen molecule called a free radical.

This was the dawn of research into antioxidants and free radicals. Searching for ways to fight these free radicals has been the source of intense interest among scientists who want to find ways to improve and extend life. The enormous market for products that will help our bodies neutralize these dangerous free radicals has also resulted in claims by supplement makers that aren't always born out by the facts. Pills, powders, oils, foods, and beverages all make claims and counterclaims about their powers as antioxidants.

No one disputes the immense damage caused by free radicals.

These unstable oxygen molecules produce what is called oxidative stress, which has now been linked to more than one hundred diseases. Search the medical literature on oxidative stress, and you will find more than 39,000 papers. What's more, free radicals and the resulting oxidative stress have been linked to aging, which is why I am including them in this book.

Back in 1969, when McCord and Fridovich published their groundbreaking findings on superoxide dismutase in the *Journal of Biological Chemistry*, their paper was met largely with indifference, even in the field. McCord remembers presenting the findings for the first time to his peers at the Federation of American Societies for Experimental Biology in Atlantic City, New Jersey. He talked about this remarkable antioxidant enzyme that scavenges free radicals.

"Almost everyone's response was, 'What's a free radical?' " recalls McCord, who is now a professor of medicine at the University of Colorado Health Sciences Center and works for a supplement maker.

There are different markers of oxidative stress in the body that increase more or less in a straight line as we age. Your level at forty is greater than your level at thirty. Your level at fifty is greater than your level at forty, and so on. Oxidative stress is like the wear and tear on a car, McCord says. In fact, one way to view aging is the slow oxidation of your body. This raises a question: What, if anything, can we do to stop free radicals in our bodies from oxidizing—or aging—us in order to extend our lives and improve our health? Before I look at that question, let's consider what we mean when we talk about antioxidants.

FIGHTING FREE RADICALS

Many of the systems in our body exist simply to take in oxygen and get it to our cells. We breathe oxygen into our lungs, transfer it to our red blood cells, and then our heart pumps it around our bodies, where cells use it to burn sugars to create energy. Unfortunately, there is a downside to this process. A byproduct of this energy production is an unstable form of the oxygen molecule. This is a free radical, and it can wreak havoc at the cellular level, damaging cells. That means oxygen, the same basic element that sustains us, may sew the seeds of cellular aging. Extending the car analogy, McCord likens these free radicals to incomplete combustion in a car's engine. In a car, the result is the production of carbon monoxide.

Unlike a car, we have built-in ways to repair minor damage and neutralize free radicals: antioxidants. They are able to scavenge most of these free radicals. However, they do not get all of them, and as we age, the remaining free radicals cause damage. Our own "engine" becomes less efficient. The "tailpipe emissions" get dirtier. These dirty emissions, the free radicals, eventually cause too much damage to be repaired by the body's own mechanisms. As a result, our bodies start breaking down.

Ground zero for oxidative damage is the mitochondria, the cells' power plants. Mitochondria are microscopic, sausage-shaped structures inside the cells. Hundreds of mitochondria exist in every cell. The mitochondria convert sugars and oxygen into adenosine triphosphate (ATP), an energy-releasing molecule that powers most of what goes on in the cell.

Like most power plants, the process is not perfectly efficient. There is some "pollution." In the case of the mitochondria, the potentially harmful by-products are the free radicals. The free-radical oxygen molecules are highly reactive because they are missing one electron, and electrons are most stable when they're paired. To become more stable, free radicals steal electrons from other molecules. These molecules, in turn, become unstable and steal molecules from still other molecules. The chain reaction results in cellular damage, including damage to DNA and the mitochondria themselves. Damage to the DNA can cause tumors and cancer. Damage to the mitochondria causes them to become less efficient and, over time, generate less energy-producing ATP and more free radicals. Eventually, enough oxidative damage occurs to trigger the cell to self-destruct. As oxidative damage accumulates, it can damage connective and nerve tissues and blood vessels.

Energy production in our cells is not the only reason free radicals form in our bodies. Smoking, exposure to the sun, and other environmental factors also produce free radicals that can cause premature cellular aging.

It stands to reason that anything we can do to eliminate free radicals would greatly benefit us in our quest to live longer, healthier lives. So it shouldn't come as a surprise that our bodies have developed ways to fight rampaging free radicals. Vitamins A, C, and E, SOD, and two other enzymes you probably haven't heard of—catalase and glutathione peroxidase—prevent most but not all of the oxidative damage in cells. As I mentioned earlier, oxidative damage still takes place. Stopping that process could be one of the biggest keys to chasing life. How can we better arm our bodies' own defenses to fight more successfully against these free radicals?

For years, researchers thought the solution might lie in antioxidant vitamins. Supplementing our diets with these vitamins, scientists reasoned, might reduce the number of free radicals and help prevent age-related diseases, such as cancer and heart disease. The government and others underwrote large-scale, long-term studies to see whether increased doses of vitamin E, vitamin A, and vitamin C would offer extra disease-fighting protection. The experiments did not produce the hoped-for results.

"I think we unfortunately went down the garden path," McCord says. "We had the idea that more would be better, and there was very little evidence of that."

The American Heart Association released a science advisory in 2004 that said research on vitamin C, vitamin E, and beta-carotene (a form of vitamin A) supplements failed to justify their use to prevent or treat cardiovascular disease. The American Cancer Society also does not advocate taking these vitamins as supplements, because the results of studies testing their results against cancer have been disappointing. In fact, in cancer patients, taking vitamin E might hurt the body's natural ability to fight tumor cells by actually helping keep tumor cells alive.

Jeffrey Blumberg, director of the Antioxidants Research Laboratory at the USDA Human Nutrition Research Center on Aging, at Tufts University, was not surprised by the studies' disappointing results and is critical of studies that look for a single nutrient, such as vitamin E, to prevent cancer or heart disease. The antioxidant defense network is complicated, he says, involving both what we eat and what our cells produce.

"It's not a one nutrient, one disease sort of thing. It's complex." Studies of the disease-fighting power of different vitamins tend to be overly simplistic, he says, trying to cure one disease with one supplement at one dose. Antioxidants work in concert, he says, as part of a dynamic system in the body.

Like the American Heart Association and American Cancer Society, Blumberg advocates a balanced diet rich in whole grains and a variety of fruits and vegetables. As we've seen, eating fruits and vegetables, which are loaded with antioxidants, has been linked to a lower risk for many chronic and potentially life-shortening diseases.

"I do feel there is an enormous power to nutrition," Blumberg says, adding that we need to eat in moderation and eat a wide array of fruits and vegetables to maximize the power of good nutrition. "You need that diversity, that variety of plant foods to provide the full complement of antioxidant nutrients."

McCord, now in the Division of Pulmonary Sciences and Critical Care Medicine at the University of Colorado Health Sciences Center, is not ready to give up on using supplements as antioxidants just yet. The biochemist thinks the disappointments from vitamin studies do not show that antioxidant supplements do not work, just that the research has been misdirected.

"Antioxidant therapy is by no means a dead topic; we have simply been looking at the wrong ones," McCord says. The focus, he says, should be on how we can supplement our diets to increase the levels of the two enzymes that do the heavy lifting when it comes to neutralizing free radicals: superoxide dismutase (SOD), the enzyme he codiscovered almost four decades ago, and catalase. These two enzymes, he says, are responsible for scavenging 99 percent of the free radicals in the body. If we can get the body to produce more of these enzymes, he reasons, then it would do a better job at fighting free radicals. Don't bother popping pills containing SOD. This is useless, because it is digested and churned up by the stomach like any other protein.

McCord says there are about forty plants, most of them used in traditional medicine in India and China, that have been shown to induce the body to produce more SOD and catalase. McCord recently coauthored an article in the journal *Free Radical Biology and Medicine* that showed how a supplement containing five such plant extracts not only increased the body's production of SOD and catalase but decreased the markers for oxidative stress associated with aging. Whether this translates into longer life remains to be seen. The supplement contained extracts of the following:

1. green tea
2. turmeric

3. milk thistle
4. ashwaganda and
5. bacopa.

Ashwaganda (also spelled ashwagandha) is a plant also known as winter cherry. Bacopa is an herb. This was a very small study, with only twenty-nine participants, but statistically very strong. Still a lot more research needs to be done.

"It may not be the final answer, but it may open a doorway that has a lot of answers behind it," says McCord. He enjoys thinking that the enzyme he discovered almost forty years ago may be at the heart of antioxidant research in the years to come.

BUYERS BEWARE

Of course, supplements are not limited to antioxidants, and increasingly, Americans have been turning to them to cure what ails them, looking for help for everything from weight loss and sore joints to depression and diabetes. I suspect the rise in popularity of herbal medicine coincides to some degree with a growing dissatisfaction with modern medicine, which is too bad.

In any event, millions of Americans now take supplements; estimates range from 15 percent to 40 percent of the population. Even President Bush reportedly takes supplements. Annual supplement sales in the United States now top $20 billion, yet the industry is largely unregulated.

Unlike prescription drugs, supplements do not require approval from the Food and Drug Administration (FDA). Because supplements are derived from natural ingredients, many people assume they are inherently safe. Most of the 29,000 supplements on the market are, but there are no guarantees and little government supervision—at least in the United States. Also, there are no guarantees about the concentration and purity of supplements on the market. Some have been found to contain prescription medication to boost their efficacy. Others have contained toxic heavy metals.

Even when the supplements themselves are safe and reliable, they can cause medical problems if they are not used correctly or if they are taken in large doses. Supplements also have the potential for dangerous interactions with drugs, a real danger, considering the huge number of Americans who take prescription medicine. Certainly, you should consult your doctor before taking any supplements, especially if you are already taking any prescription medicine.

I was amazed to learn that even when a supplement is dangerous, the federal government has trouble banning it. Under the 1994 law governing supplements, federal regulators must prove supplements unsafe, not the other way around. In 2004, the FDA attempted to ban the diet supplement ephedra after it was linked to heart attack, stroke, high blood pressure, and at least 164 deaths. A federal judge overturned the ban, ruling that the federal government could not issue a blanket ban on the supplement, but needed to state which dosages were unsafe.

Supplement makers also do not have to report adverse reactions to their products, as drug companies do. The federal government estimates only about 1 percent of adverse reactions are reported, despite a hotline and Web site set up to record such reports. More than one in eight calls to the California Poison Control Center was prompted by a child's adverse reaction to a dietary supplement, including vomiting, nausea, and increased heart rate, the *Los Angeles Times* reported.

Shining the light on one potentially harmful supplement does not prevent other potentially dangerous supplements from filling the void in the marketplace. For example, when the dangers of ephedra became known, a supplement made from bitter orange peel, *Citrus aurantium*, was advertised as an ephedra-free alternative for dieters and athletes. However, *Citrus aurantium* may pose many of the same risks as ephedra, according to a research review published in the journal *Experimental Biology and Medicine*.

Many companies that produce supplements suggest they are safe because they have been used for thousands of years or are derived from ancient medicine. Being natural or part of a traditional treatment does not make it safe. Aristolochic acid, derived from a Chinese herb, was sold for a variety of ailments, but turned out to be a carcinogen linked to kidney failure and death. The supplements chaparral, comfrey, germander, and kava have also been linked to liver damage and death. None of these cautionary tales has slowed the booming market for dietary supplements.

Echinacea and the Common Cold

The best selling of these is echinacea, an extract from the coneflower, which is a member of the sunflower family. An estimated 15 million Americans take echinacea to prevent and treat colds. There is little clinical evidence it does either. A 2005 study funded by the federal government and published in the *New England Journal of Medicine* found none of three different preparations of echinacea on the market were successful at preventing the cold. Supporters of echinacea said the dose tested was too low. Other government-funded studies found echinacea did not work as a treatment for the common cold in adults or for upper respiratory tract infections in children. Nonetheless, the National Center for Complementary and Alternative Medicine is continuing to fund the study of echinacea as a possible treatment for upper respiratory infections.

Supplement takers, including Laura Brown, reading the preceding paragraphs will no doubt conclude that I have been somehow coopted or brainwashed by some medical-pharmaceutical industrial complex. My response is that I believe in the scientific method, and if a well-run trial shows a treatment does not work any better than a placebo, we should first try to replicate the results and then think twice about continuing that course of treatment.

Still, I doubt anything I write here will dissuade anyone of the efficacy of echinacea or any other supplement. To be sure, belief alone is a powerful healing tool, which I will take up in detail in chapter 8.

Let's consider some of the other popular dietary supplements, such as garlic. The lower rate of heart disease among southern Europeans, who eat the garlic-rich Mediterranean diet, has led to a lot of interest in the plant. An estimated 7 million Americans use garlic supplements. Three dozen clinical trials in adults have found that taking various garlic preparations resulted in a small but statistically significant reduction in total cholesterol over the short term. Studies show garlic also may protect against platelet aggregation, which can raise the risk of stroke. Few studies have looked at the efficacy of fresh garlic, although research suggests heating garlic right after it is crushed or chopped appears to diminish garlic's beneficial properties. Some scientists recommend letting crushed or chopped garlic sit for ten minutes before cooking with it. Several population studies suggest garlic and other vegetables in its class, such as onions and leeks, may help protect against cancer.

Saint-John's-wort, a long-lived plant with yellow flowers, has been used for centuries as an herbal treatment for depression. An estimated 1.5 million Americans take Saint-John's-wort supplements. There is some evidence Saint-John's-wort works to treat mild to moderate depression, but studies have concluded the supplement does not work to treat more severe depression.

Consuming the root of the Asian ginseng plant is said to improve overall health, increase mental and physical performance, lower blood sugar, and control blood sugar. It should come as no surprise, then, that drinks and other products add ginseng to attract health-conscious consumers. Does it work? Some studies have concluded ginseng may lower blood sugar and boost immune function. According to the National Center for Complementary and Alternative Medicine, the research has not been conclusive.

Gingko biloba is another supplement added to various beverages. It has long been touted as a memory-boosting supplement. However, research suggests it does not improve memory as advertised.

Soy products are also popular supplements, reputed to be heart healthy and protective against prostate and breast cancers. Proponents point to the Japanese and others in Asia who eat soy-rich diets and have far fewer cases of these cancers than their counterparts in much of the West. No clinical evidence currently supports the assertion that soy lowers the risk for these hormone-related cancers. Studies do suggest soy products offer moderate benefits in lowering LDL ("bad") cholesterol and triglycerides.

Let's consider the supplements President Bush is known to take. First, he takes a daily multivitamin. The president also takes a combination of glucosamine and chondroitin and a fish oil supplement. Glucosamine and chondroitin are taken for joint pain. President Bush suffers from knee pain from years of jogging, something he forgoes now in favor of riding a mountain bike or using an elliptical machine.

A government study found glucosamine and chondroitin together did not provide significant relief for most knee pain, compared to a placebo. The two widely used supplements also failed when tested separately. However, the supplements did bring relief for participants with moderate to severe pain, according to the large-scale study. President Bush had knee surgery in 1997 on his left knee, so it's quite possible he fits in this moderate to severe group.

How about the other supplement President Bush reportedly takes—fish oil? Fish oil contains omega-3 fatty acids. A review of the medical literature suggests eating fish or taking a fish oil supplement can reduce the risk of heart attack and heart disease, though fish oil alone did not affect cholesterol levels. Omega-3 fatty acids are also thought to be good for the brain. Have you ever heard the old mantra that fish is brain food? Clinical evidence is not yet strong enough to make any conclusions about whether this is the case, but a number of doctors believe it does help protect the brain against Alzheimer's and other problems. No doubt more and better studies will be conducted in coming years to see if fish and fish oil really do keep our brains healthier. Incidentally, if you are looking for other ways to keep the brain sharp, I'll have more on that in chapter 5.

EAT YOUR SUPPLEMENTS

Blumberg, at Tufts, is not a big fan of supplements. He is a staunch believer in a diet consisting of a healthy variety of foods, eaten in moderation. But he is not ready to write off supplements entirely. Blumberg sees times when supplements can be beneficial and fill a void in our diets.

For instance, consider the person in the process of shifting from an unhealthy diet to a healthy diet. Old eating habits need to be discarded. New ones need to be developed. No one makes the shift from junk food to healthy food overnight. During the transition, supplements are a good way to make up for nutritional shortfalls, Blumberg says. But he is quick to add, "Dietary supplements are not dietary substitutes." In the long run, it is always best to make a change in diet, but if there is no chance you are going to get enough of a certain nutrient in your diet in the short term, you should take a supplement. Shortfalls are common for most people, and a typical multivitamin/multimineral can help fill the gap between actual intakes and requirements.

There is another time when taking a supplement makes sense, Blumberg says. There is a chance you realistically are not going to eat certain foods that contain a vital nutrient. You may intensely dislike the taste of fish, for example. In this case, taking an omega-3 supplement makes sense. It also makes sense to eat foods fortified with vitamins and nutrients if that helps you achieve recommended levels of different vitamins and nutrients.

As I mentioned in the previous chapter, most Americans are falling short of the recommended daily allowances of vitamins A, C, and E and the minerals calcium, magnesium, and potassium. This certainly seems to suggest many could benefit from a multivitamin with minerals.

Other Americans, it appears, take too many vitamins. Some doctors believe many are popping vitamins to counteract unhealthy diets and lifestyles, with some potentially dangerous side effects.

Also, almost half of all Americans take some prescription medicine. For older Americans, the percentage is higher. Drugs may change the way your body metabolizes food, which may result in nutrients being flushed from the body or less well absorbed. This, too, would be a good reason to take supplements.

Finally, as we get older, we need more of certain nutrients to maintain healthy levels, and this too may require supplements. For example, as we age, we become less efficient at converting sunlight into vitamin D. As a result, we need to include more foods with vitamin D in our diet, such as milk, which is fortified with vitamin D, or we need to take a vitamin supplement.

Also, vitamin B_{12} and folic acid are less well absorbed by the elderly, who don't secrete as much hydrochloric acid in the stomach. The result is a higher stomach pH (less acidity) and the reduced ability to absorb these nutrients. Vitamin B_6 requirements in the elderly also go up, although experts are not sure why. It's possible it is utilized more rapidly. All this happens at a time in life when appetite decreases for many, meaning there is less opportunity to make up this potential nutritional shortfall.

Too little calcium will result in a loss in bone density and osteoporosis, but should we take calcium supplements? A seven-year study involving 36,000 women, published in 2006 in the *New England Journal of Medicine*, upended conventional wisdom by concluding that seven years of taking calcium and vitamin D supplements daily provided minimal protection against broken bones for older women. As a result of the study, a number of doctors and nutritionists concluded that women with low bone density should take medicine to help build bone mass. Several drugs are available. Osteoporosis affects about 10 million Americans, mostly women, and leads to 1.5 million fractures a year. If you are worried about the strength of your bones, you can have a bone density scan, a painless type of X-ray.

Women (and men) who do not have bone density issues should try to get their daily calcium requirement through their diet. The National Institutes of Health's (NIH's) Office of Dietary Supplements recommends two or three servings a day of calcium-rich foods. Examples of servings are 1 cup of milk, 8 ounces of yogurt, or 1.5 ounces of natural cheese, such as cheddar. Orange juice also comes fortified with calcium. Most Americans do not get enough calcium in what they eat and drink, which is why the National Osteoporosis Foundation continues to advocate calcium supplements for most Americans, despite the disappointing results of the large-scale study mentioned above.

Experts warn that osteoporosis begins early. Because we build 90 percent of our bone mass by age nineteen, young people should be encouraged to get enough calcium in their diets. Children allowed to choose sodas over milk as they mature may be setting themselves up for a fall later in life, quite literally.

HORMONE REPLACEMENT

As we age, our body chemistry changes. Production of hormones such as testosterone and human growth hormone declines. Replacing these and other hormones to more youthful levels in an effort to extend vitality is controversial and potentially dangerous. That doesn't mean there isn't a lot of interest.

Open up Google and search for "human growth hormone," and you'll get more than 5 million hits. Human growth hormone (HGH) is produced by the pituitary gland and spurs bone and tissue growth. Between the ages of twenty and sixty, the levels of HGH released by the gland drop by half or more. Now a growing number of doctors appear willing to prescribe the hormone as an antiaging therapy.

Some people are born with a pituitary gland that does not produce enough HGH. This results is dwarfism, the treatment of which was the hormone's original medicinal use. HGH was discovered fifty years ago and was originally harvested from cadavers. Twenty years ago, researchers figured out how to make it synthetically. Promoters of giving HGH to the aging now claim injections of the hormone will do everything from boosting muscle, memory, and sexual function to lowering blood pressure and reducing fat. The treatment can cost more than $10,000 a year.

A 1990 study of HGH in 12 older men, published in the *New England Journal of Medicine*, found the hormone reduced fat and increased muscle and bone density. A larger study in 2002, involving 125 older men and women, found HGH injections resulted in less fat and more muscle, but not increased strength.

The earlier study has been quoted extensively on the Internet, prompting the journal to post on its Web site a warning about the potentially misleading ads online.

Critics say the risks of using HGH far outweigh the potential gains. They include headaches, carpal tunnel syndrome, swelling joints, bloating, the increased risk of diabetes, and possibly tumor growth. Ironically, it may also speed the aging process. Mice with too much growth hormone die younger. The long-term risks in humans are not known, but critics say too much HGH could potentially shorten the life span of those taking it.

Testosterone is another hormone whose production peaks early in adulthood. Replacing the hormone to more youthful levels has been touted as a way to promote heart health and retain muscle mass, memory, and sex drive in men, but in large doses, it can cause hair loss and mood problems. Also, it may increase LDL, or "bad" cholesterol, and raise the risk for certain cancers, heart disease, and stroke. Some scientists have implicated testosterone as the culprit behind men's shorter life expectancy. Women who take testosterone to counteract menopause may start exhibiting male secondary sex traits, such as hairiness.

Promoters of hormone treatments to improve vitality also crow about the benefits of thyroid hormones and an adrenal hormone called dehydroepiandrosterone, or DHEA. Production peaks in the midtwenties and then decreases as we age. Not much is known about what happens if we bring the levels back to where they were when we were younger. Possible problems with supplementing thyroid hormones include heart arrhythmias and bone loss, while DHEA may cause liver damage and breast enlargement in men and hairiness in women.

The Search for Eternal Youth

Rejuvenating hormone therapies are not new. More than a century ago, the French physiologist Charles-Édouard Brown-Séquard thought he had discovered the secret to eternal youth in the testicles of animals. At seventy-two, he removed and crushed dog and guinea pig testes, testicular blood, and seminal fluid, mixed them with water, and injected the filtered extract under the skin of his own arm. After three weeks of injections, Brown-Séquard reported greater strength, mental concentration, and stamina. More than twelve thousand physicians injected thousands of doses of similar concoctions, named Sequarine and billed as "the medicine of the future," into the general public. An ad for the serum claimed it "embodies the very essence of animal energy" and was successful in treating a long list of ailments, including nervousness, rheumatism, gout, diabetes, paralysis, and influenza. Of course, Sequarine was no age-defying potion, and the fad eventually faded.

It's too soon to say whether HGH and some of the other hormone therapies being prescribed today will succumb to the same fate. Not enough research has been done on the long-term effects of HGH and other antiaging hormone treatments to prove their safety and efficacy. Given the number of people willing to take chances with their health by replacing hormones that naturally decline with age, we will get more telling answers about their long-term effects on the body in the years to come. In the meantime, it seems at least premature to begin injections or other treatments with these hormones.

UNLIKELY ELIXIRS

History is filled with dietary antidotes to aging, most of them unappetizing or downright bizarre. Chinese Taoists thought eating foods related to long-lived plants and animals would help increase longevity. They recommended crane's eggs, tortoise soup, and the products of pines and cypresses. The thirteenth-century English philosopher and scientist Roger Bacon, no doubt looking at the wrinkled skin of the elderly, concluded that the loss of "innate moisture" over time caused old age. He advocated taking baths and ingesting small quantities of pearl, coral, aloe wood, gold, and "bone from a stag's heart." These were intended to replace "innate moisture" lost through aging. The breath of a virgin was also recommended for old men, who would absorb some of the "vital principle" by being in the company of youth.

I'm not going to advocate dining on stag's heart, but there are potential health benefits to be found in some unlikely places. Take dark chocolate, for example. Eating dark chocolate boosts the blood's antioxidant power by 20 percent, according to research published in a paper in *Nature*. The antioxidant in chocolate is called epicatechin. Milk chocolate is much less effective. A study of older men in the Netherlands found eating the equivalent of a third of a chocolate bar a day may lower blood pressure and the risk of death. Dark chocolate (but not milk chocolate or white chocolate) also appears to inhibit the aggregation of platelets, an early step in the formation of blood clots that can cause heart attack or stroke. Cocoa beans contain flavonoids. Red wine; apples; berries; and green, white, black, and oolong teas also contain flavonoids, which are thought to increase nitric oxide in the blood and improve the function of blood vessels. However, chocolate also contains sugar and fat, so while a little chocolate may be a good thing, a lot of chocolate may be too much of a good thing.

How about red wine? Much has been written about the potential life-extending properties of red wine, thanks to the so-called French paradox—the relatively low level of heart disease in France despite the prevalence of high-fat foods and cigarette smoking. The French also drink a lot of red wine, leading to speculation that a compound in the wine, resveratrol, may be responsible. Resveratrol is a compound that shows antioxidant, anti-inflammatory, and potentially artery friendly properties in laboratory and animal studies. In addition to wine, resveratrol is found in red grapes, red grape juice, peanuts, blueberries, and cranberries. All wines contain resveratrol, though red wines contain more than whites or rosés. In cells cultured outside the body, resveratrol inhibited the spread of a number of human cancers. Resveratrol has also increased by 60 percent the life spans of yeast, flies, nematodes, and a short-lived fish native to Zimbabwe. It's not known whether resveratrol has life-extending properties in humans.

Green tea has achieved a sort of cult status for its reputed health-giving properties. It's so "hot," it's included in sodas and other drinks. As I mentioned earlier, an extract of green tea was in the antioxidant supplement the University of Colorado's McCord tested with some success. Teas, including green tea, have been shown to lower cancer risk in some animal studies, but population studies in people have not been conclusive.

How about coffee? Many people drink coffee not to become healthier but to give them a caffeine-fueled boost. Still, University of California, Davis researchers think brewed coffee (both caffeinated and decaf) has the same amount of antioxidant as three oranges. A number of studies also suggests that coffee lowers the risk for type 2 diabetes, Parkinson's disease (for men), and possibly colorectal cancer. Not all the news about coffee is good, however. Caffeine raises blood pressure, which can be dangerous for people with hypertension. Unfiltered coffee, such as espresso and French press, also increases cholesterol. Filtered coffee doesn't have much of an effect on cholesterol. Before you run off on a coffee binge, remember that as with most things, moderation is key.

EDUCATE YOURSELF

If you are excited about the idea of taking herbs and supplements as a way of taking responsibility for your health, know that there are a lot of claims being made that need to be checked. Educate yourself. Remember that snake oil salesmen have been boasting about the healing properties of all sorts of things for centuries. We want to believe them because we want more control over our well-being. Remember, too, that just because a substance is "natural" and has been around for centuries, it is not necessarily safe. Laura Brown has taken this important first step toward controlling her own health. While the scientific data may not support her decisions, there is no arguing that she believes these supplements work for her. She has 45 million Americans alone who agree with her. If you are one of them or are thinking of becoming one of them, refer to this chapter, and do your homework.

This chapter has attempted to use clinical data to cut through the claims made about some of the more popular supplements. There are thousands of supplement makers out there, some of them making exuberant promises about their products. Don't take their word for it. The NIH's Office of Dietary Supplements Web site has a lot of information that can help you make informed decisions. So do the Web sites of the Mayo Clinic and Oregon State University's Linus Pauling Institute. Finally, remember that there are no miracle cures. As you chase the healthiest possible life, be smart about what you put in your body. Next stop: run for your life, because there are no shortcuts or substitutes for hard work.

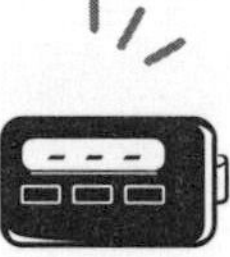

Paging Dr. Gupta

- ✓ There is no fountain of youth. Beware the product that says it will make you younger.
- ✓ Go to the source, not the supplement. There is no substitute for a diet filled with fruits and vegetables.
- ✓ Stay away from human growth hormone. The potential for harm outweighs any potential benefit.
- ✓ Depending on your age, your race, and where you live, you might consider taking a vitamin D supplement.
- ✓ Discover the unlikely elixirs. Dark chocolate, red wine, and coffee may extend life.
- ✓ Just because something is natural, it is not guaranteed to be safe.

CHAPTER 4

Run for Your Life

As an Allstate executive for nearly forty years, James Hammond was always on the move. While his industry transformed itself, he relocated from one southern state to another, training the future generation of managers in the insurance industry. In all, he lived in ten different states during his career. Hammond reminds me of most of my patients. It's not that he was a couch potato by any means. In fact, he was quite active; but he was simply too busy to really exercise. Occasionally on the weekends, he would get in a jog. If this sounds familiar, it should. Hammond represents the vast majority of working-class adults around the world. Like you and me, they have the best intentions, but fitness takes a progressively lower priority as they get older. Hammond's life, however, took a wildly divergent turn. In fact, though he never competed in an organized sport in his entire life, he decided to take it up—at the age of eighty-six! It was then that a friend suggested he enter the Georgia Golden

Olympics. He did it and started down a remarkable path of continued good health.

Hammond decided to enter the state games in the 100-meter dash and, to his surprise, won a gold medal with a time of 30 seconds. It's a time Hammond in his own affable way now laughs off as "very slow." Still, he was hooked and was inspired to start running seriously. His goal was to get his time down to 18 or 19 seconds so he could place in the National Senior Games the following year in Baton Rouge, Louisiana.

Training on his own, Hammond was able to get his time down to 23 seconds by "running and running and running," but he could get no faster.

"I was ready to throw in the towel," Hammond recalls. Finally, someone recommended getting a coach. Hammond approached the man, a schoolteacher who had been a sprinter at Louisiana State University. He agreed to work with Hammond only if the octogenarian wanted to win. Hammond assured him he did.

Hammond's training went to the next level. He began lifting weights to build up strength in addition to running hard. His times started dropping. Every week, his coach would drive him to an open track meet at the University of Florida in Tallahassee. He broke 20 seconds, then 19. The day before the nationals, he competed in the meet and clocked an 18.4. The next day, he ran an 18.3 in Baton Rouge and won the silver medal. Hammond says the only reason he didn't win the gold was he ignored a piece of last-minute advice from his coach to pay no attention to the other runners. Halfway through the race, Hammond noticed he was out in front and eased up, convinced he had the race won. Winning the silver only fueled his drive to work harder.

Hammond has since moved to the Minneapolis area, where he lives within 8 miles of his only child, a minister; his three grandchildren, and six great-grandchildren. Every day, you can find him at a local health club, lifting weights, running a variety of sprints and other distances, and stretching.

"I know it helps to walk and jog, but I'm convinced what keeps your body working is strenuous exercise," Hammond says. He speaks often to his peers and those seniors who are decades younger on the benefits of fitness.

As the next National Senior Games approached, in Richmond in 2003, Hammond was convinced he would win the gold medal. A day before the race, though, he decided to buy track cleats to help his time. During the race, a spike caught in the track surface, and Hammond was pitched face-first onto the track. He left the meet in an ambulance, with a broken wrist.

"It was a near-fatal blow to my ego," he jokes. The disappointment only made him more determined. "The worst things in life can be real character builders. I come from a family that preached the power of positive thinking. My mother liked to say things like, 'You'll find good if you look for it.' "

Hammond says he inherited his positive attitude from his

mother and father. His longevity, though, he credits to his fitness regimen, not genetics.

"My mother died when she was forty-nine. My dad died when he was sixty-five. I had a grandmother that made it to ninety-one and a great-grandfather that made it to ninety-one. Outside of those two, not many lived past their eighties."

Now at ninety-two, not only is he alive, he is a world-class sprinter, a national record holder with his eye on the world mark.

"It helps every aspect of your life. It's not possible to enjoy life if you're not in good health, and I'm in perfect health," Hammond says.

"It's been a wonderful thing for me. Exercise has extended my good health through my eighties into my nineties. I'm in as good shape now as I was ten to fifteen years ago. I've really loved it. It's opened up a whole new world for me. It's made my eighties and nineties some of the happiest years of my life," Hammond says.

Hammond has plenty of company. Even as America's collective girth grows, there is a parallel fitness boom, persuading millions of Americans to challenge themselves physically.

For example, some 6.2 million Americans exercised with personal trainers in 2004, up 55 percent in five years, according to the International Health, Racquet & Sportsclub Association.

Also, the number of marathoners finishing races increased from 120,000 in 1980 to 423,000 in 2004, according to Running USA, a national trade organization for the sport of distance running. The number of men finishing marathons more than doubled during that period. The number of women increased fourteenfold! Road races, too, have experienced a remarkable growth in popularity, from 1 million finishers in 1980 to 8 million finishers in 2005.

Even triathlons, the often-grueling swimming, biking, and running races, have experienced enormous growth. The number of people joining USA Triathlon, the governing body for the sport, more than tripled from 2000 through mid-2006 to 66,000. Even more impressive, the number of competitors in Ironman triathlons in the United States hit a record 10,000 in 2005 and continues to grow. These are definitely not for the faint of heart. An Ironman USA triathlon consists of a 2.4-mile swim, a 112-mile bike ride, and a marathon.

What James Hammond and many others are teaching us is that aging does not always spell the end to fast times and extreme fitness—even for the most serious competitors. Former Northwestern University swimmer Richard T. Abrahams became the first fifty-year-old to break 50 seconds in the 100-yard freestyle. His time at age fifty was faster than when he competed at the 1964 Olympic Trials. A decade later, in 2005, Abrahams became the first sixty-year-old to break 50 seconds in the 100-yard freestyle. His best time during those intervening ten years actually slowed by only 0.34 seconds.

The Ukrainian Tatyana Pozdnyakova won the 2003 City of Los Angeles Marathon at age forty-eight. The Los Angeles

Marathon is not some small-time affair. It attracts elite runners from around the world. Pozdnyakova finished more than three minutes ahead of the second female finisher in the highly competitive field. What's more, Pozdnyakova won the Los Angeles Marathon again the next year, at forty-nine.

"I don't think about age," she told a newspaper reporter. "My age is very high, but my head is strong. It is not about your body. It is discipline."

EXERCISE MORE, AGE LESS

As I was traveling the country talking to people about this book, one thing started to become increasingly clear. While so many of us are in search of the magical shortcut to boosting our life expectancy, we don't take nearly enough advantage of what we already know. As a result of what I have learned, I have already started to change and lengthen my life. Here is one example that is almost guaranteed to increase your life span. As we grow older, we tend to lose lung capacity, flexibility, and strength. The fittest among us will gradually become slower, weaker, and less flexible. But that's for people starting at their peak. Most of us are not there. Most of us are not even close. That means we can actually become biologically "younger" by getting into better shape. Think about that for a second. No pills, surgery, or magic potions, and you can still make yourself . . . younger. As we've already seen with James Hammond, you can become quicker, stronger, and more flexible if you really work at it.

Let's consider the shape most Americans are in right now. More than two-thirds of American adults are clinically overweight. Not surprisingly, six in ten Americans surveyed said they never participate in any vigorous, leisure time physical activity.

You don't have to be a hard-core swimmer like Abrahams, a distance runner like Pozdnyakova, or a sprinting nonagenarian like Hammond to reap the benefits of exercise. Lifting weights, walking, riding a bike, and jogging can all help the heart and lungs.

A study published in the *Journal of the American College of Cardiology* found much of the decline in exercise capacity as we get older is not from an aging cardiovascular system but largely from the result of plain and simple inactivity. Sedentary seniors who underwent a six-month exercise program of walking or jogging, bicycling, and stretching were able to improve their efficiency at sending oxygen to working muscles to levels closer to twenty- and thirty-year-olds. Put simply, they were able to do a lot more without becoming exhausted.

Walk for Health

Another study, conducted by researchers at the University of Pittsburgh School of Public Health, found that the ability of people seventy to seventy-nine to walk a quarter mile was a significant predictor of death and poor health. Those who could walk the distance—one lap on a standard track—were much more likely to be alive six years later. More than that, it forecasted how much disability and illness they were likely to have in the coming six years.

Lifting weights, too, should not be overlooked. Strength training can help reduce the symptoms of a number of diseases and chronic conditions, such as diabetes, obesity, back pain, depression, and arthritis. It can also boost metabolism by 15 percent. A Tufts University study put older men and women with moderate to severe osteoarthritis on a sixteen-week strength-training program, and their pain decreased by 43 percent. I was amazed at how much the simple bench press can do to increase your life span. This exercise alone will open up the ribs and the chest cavity. That, in turn, gives our lungs more room and makes us less prone to pneumonia as we get older. This is critically important, because respiratory disease becomes an increasing concern as we get older. In fact, every expert I spoke with recommended an upper body resistance-training program for men and women. That one exercise alone, because of its ability to ward off pneumonia later in life, can add years and help us chase life like no other.

Also, don't forget exercises to strengthen your back muscles. So much of our lives are spent hunched over computers, the back is stressed like it's been at no other time in human history. And let's not forget the obvious. Weight lifting can build muscle mass and strength. Strength training can also increase flexibility, improve balance, preserve bone density, and prevent osteoporosis, which affects an estimated 8 million women in the United States. A study on postmenopausal women found lifting weights twice a week resulted in a 75 percent increase in strength, 13 percent increase in balance, and 1 percent increase in hip and spine bone density. Bone density may not sound like such a big deal, but consider this: the broken hip is the number-one cause for institutionalizing the elderly in nursing homes. By avoiding broken bones, the elderly stand a much better chance of leading independent or more independent lives.

THE BASICS

If you are just starting out, you should consult your doctor before beginning any exercise program. You might consider hiring a trainer at a gym to show you how the equipment works and how much weight you should be lifting on each machine. In general, you should find a weight that you can lift eight to twelve times using good form, and then, two minutes later, do another set. If you can handle more than twelve repetitions on each set, you should consider increasing the weight. If you can not lift the weight eight times on one of the sets, you should consider decreasing the weight.

If you are just starting out and prefer to lift at home instead of a gym, buy two small hand weights. You can do bicep curls and overhead presses with them. You can use the wall for "wall push-ups." You can also use the steps in your home to build your quadriceps by stepping up with one leg and then the other. Holding the back of a chair, raising one leg at a time to the side, is also a good exercise to begin a fitness routine.

Warm up before you start lifting. In general, here is a good rule: Begin with the large muscle groups and work your way to the smaller ones. When you lift, it should be a smooth, fluid motion, not a violent heave. You can count to four as you lift the weight, if you'd like, to make sure you are not rushing it. Don't forget to breathe. Exhale when you are lifting the weight. Inhale when you bring the weight back to the starting position. Don't forget to lower the weight slowly as well. Younger weight lifters should give each muscle group twenty-four hours to recuperate between workouts. Older lifters should double that and wait forty-eight hours before working out with the same muscle group.

Aerobic exercise can lower the risk of such chronic conditions as heart disease, diabetes, osteoporosis, and breast and colon cancer. Aerobic exercise includes walking, jogging, bike riding, swimming, yoga, Pilates—anything that gets you breathing hard and your heart rate up.

Exercise should be done three to five times per week. You should make exercise part of your routine and give it the same importance as eating or sleeping. Don't let exercise be the part of your schedule that is the first to go when there is a "fire drill" at work or a crisis at home. Think of your life as a marathon and exercise a vital part of "going the distance." You will actually be more productive at work and have more energy in your home life if you take the time to be active.

In general, physical activity is also linked to reduced stress, healthier weight, and lower cholesterol, blood sugar, and blood pressure. Exercise can also help you get a good night's sleep (as long as you're not exercising late in the day).

Get Motivated

If you are prone to procrastination or to putting off exercise, find a workout partner, join a cycling club, or sign up for an exercise boot camp. Camaraderie and peer pressure are great motivators. Giving and getting encouragement while you become fit makes exercise enjoyable—something to look forward to rather than a necessary task.

Another way to motivate yourself is to sign up for a 5K or 10K road race a month or two from now, even if you are not yet ready for one. It's a great way to get you out the door and on your way to a fitter lifestyle. Give yourself a physical goal, and you'll be amazed how a healthier diet naturally follows. Who wants to stuff themselves with junk if they have to run 10 kilometers? If you don't know how to train for a race, look on the Internet. An online search should turn up a number of different week-by-week workouts to get you ready for running just about any distance. The important thing is to raise the bar. Challenge yourself.

Even if you don't want to become a world-class nonagenarian, you can still make great strides as you get older, especially if you are a couch potato. No need for the elaborate wind sprints and other exercises Hammond puts himself through every afternoon at his gym. Most of the rest of us will benefit greatly from far simpler routines not only at the gym but in our daily lives. Next time, take the stairs instead of the elevator, or walk up the escalator instead of riding it. Find more ways to keep your body active in our largely sedentary world.

Hammond himself said his fitness routine started from scratch, so to speak, and gradually built to the intensity he now brings to his workouts. You are never too old to begin a fitness routine. Remember, Hammond didn't begin really exercising until his eighties. Of course, the earlier you start a regular exercise routine, the healthier you'll be as you age. What is most striking is the association between an active life and a longer, healthier life. Not only will your body be healthier, but your brain will be as well (more on this in chapter 5). There are very few things in medicine that have such a well-defined relationship. In addition, if you put in the time and effort, you will almost certainly be able to improve your strength, endurance, and flexibility.

Anyone who is just beginning to get in shape needs to remember to start slowly, no matter how tempting it is to begin in fourth gear. Starting out too fast is a surefire route to injury. You should also have reasonable expectations. Expecting too much, too early almost certainly guarantees disappointment. That said, it is a good idea to set specific, measurable goals. As I've mentioned, they should be reasonable. Don't set your sights to levels that are unattainable. No matter how hard I trained, I would not be able to break the four-minute mile. Goals should include how often you intend to exercise and what physical accomplishments you would like to achieve, both in the short term and long term. Physical goals may be walking for an hour or running a ten-minute mile. They may also be functional accomplishments. For example, you may want to be able to walk all eighteen holes on a golf course or be able to walk up the five flights of stairs to your office. Remember, progress will be incremental. There will not be any great leap forward in your physical abilities.

You know, as I was writing this book and hearing James Hammond's story, I felt inspired in my own way. My exercise routine had always been fairly simple and in accordance with my life. Because I have a 90-pound Weimaraner, I would run four miles every morning with him to get him in shape. I would also lift moderate weights every other day. I felt like I was pretty well conditioned, but I felt like I was punching my card instead of chasing life. So, with my newfound inspiration, I decided to sign up for a half marathon. Like Hammond, I enjoy shooting for goals. Following the same advice in this book by adding both increased aerobic training and weight training, I found my workouts to be both effective and delightful. As I ramped up my miles, my colleagues in television almost immediately told me I looked robust and younger. I finished that half marathon in under two hours, which was my aspiration, and have now made more rigorous and strenuous training a part of my life.

I did learn, though, that you should also listen to your body, especially if you are feeling pain when you exercise. If your knees are hurting when you jog, give them a break. Work out using an elliptical machine or swim. Even sixty-year-old President Bush, who has his health rated as "superior" by his doctors, had to make the switch from running seven-minute miles to riding a bicycle and using low-impact machines. Resting the joints will help. Bottom line: Don't use pain as an excuse to stop exercising. Just find new and creative ways to stay in shape.

Many people are intimidated by the gym, especially if they haven't had much exercise lately. You don't have to go to the gym to get a good workout. The Centers for Disease Control and Prevention (CDC) calculated the metabolic expenditures for various activities. What they found might surprise you. Climbing stairs was more rigorous than playing doubles tennis. Shoveling in the garden was more metabolically challenging than playing golf.

As you've probably heard, simply walking half an hour a day will do wonders for your cardiovascular health. What you may not know is that the benefits will extend beyond your heart, your lungs, and your sense of well-being. You will become healthy at the cellular level. Your mitochondria—your cells' power plants—will become stronger. Experts recommend exercise that makes you breathe harder on most or all days of the week. Assuming you have a clean bill of health, you should exercise vigorously enough so talking is difficult, but not so hard you can't talk at all.

Once you become comfortable with a basic routine, mix it up a little. Do shorter, fast walks one day and longer, slower ones the next. Try an exercise bike or an elliptical machine. A trainer I know likes to say, "Surprise your body every day."

Stretching is also vital. We naturally become less limber as we age. Only stretching will preserve our range of motion. Hammond says he works at least as hard on stretching as he does on his workouts. It's a smart decision, not only for his quest to be a world-record holder but for his general well-being. Stretching appears to have other benefits as well. Doing some light stretching before bed appears to help some people sleep. Also, yoga has been shown to reduce not only self-reported levels of stress but also levels of stress hormone in the body.

RISE UP, COUCH POTATOES

If you are one of those people who don't like even the thought of exercise, that doesn't mean you can't stay fit. There are plenty of activities that work the muscles, lungs, and heart. For example, walk instead of drive whenever possible. Instead of taking the elevator, use the stairs. Rake leaves. Garden. Dance. Ride a bike. Skip. We live in a society where everything can be incredibly easy. We can go through the day without exerting ourselves at all. We take the elevator, the escalator, the car without thinking about it.

We do it automatically. Choosing the more strenuous alternative takes a conscious decision—a new way of thinking. The next time you are standing on an escalator as it propels you to the next level, close your eyes and imagine yourself climbing a mountain instead, using every muscle group, from your tiny finger flexors to your gigantic thigh extensors. James Hammond teaches us that too many of us simply go through the routine of exercise every day. Instead of challenging our bodies with strenuous, surprising new exercises, we are content to jump on the treadmill every day, reaching a plateau in our aerobic development and never changing our metabolism or improving our core strength. If you make some simple changes, the rewards can be bountiful. Instead of suffering through his eighties and nineties plagued by inactivity and the associated diseases of the heart, lungs, and bones, Hammond was able to fill his life with steadily increasing goals and strenuous activity. Like most people who have incorporated regular fitness into their lives, Hammond never grumbled about the hard work, but instead constantly looked for ways to do even more and become even stronger. While having fun and becoming a world-class athlete in his eighties, Hammond shows us yet another way to chase life. Truth is, you don't have to start running the 100-meter dash competitively, but what can you do today to live more like James Hammond? Check out some of my best tips in the Paging Dr. Gupta box at the end of the chapter.

I realized as I traveled the world talking to people about chasing life that almost everyone had one major concern:

what is a long life without a limber mind? And that is our next stop. You are going to be amazed when I show you some simple ways to make sure your mind stays just as healthy as your body as we chase life together.

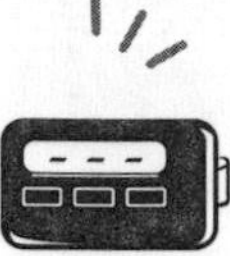

Paging Dr. Gupta

- ✓ Surprise your body every day. Try a new exercise.
- ✓ Push the limits. Chasing life is hard work. Challenge yourself with some strenuous exercise.
- ✓ Make sure to do upper-body training now. It may add years to your life.
- ✓ Stretch. Stretching should take as much time as the rest of your workout. Your body will thank you.
- ✓ Don't skip workouts, even when you're on the road.
- ✓ Exercise daily. Don't have time for a workout? Then take the stairs, park farther away, rake the leaves, or vacuum.

CHAPTER 5

Memories R Us

Chuck Ozug taught English his entire working career. He was in his classroom in Falmouth, on Cape Cod, when his heart suddenly stopped, and he collapsed. Paramedics rushed to the scene and literally brought Ozug back from the dead. Precious minutes had passed, and the lack of oxygen left Ozug with irreversible brain damage that destroyed most of his memories and prevented him from forming lasting new memories.

He now lives in a perpetual present, a frustrating, often depressing existence he counters with a quick sense of humor and a highlighter—so he can remember the passages in the newspaper he wants to show his wife, Mary Ann. He also writes poetry about his condition. One line particularly struck me: "My memory, like snowflakes, soft, faint, snowflakes soothing only for a while."

Ozug considers himself lucky he survived. Doctors at the hospital told his wife he wasn't going to make it. He says he finds joy in time spent with his wife and his two sons. Still, he lives in what he poetically describes as a never-ending blankness, often forgetting what someone has told him on the phone before he hangs up.

What is particularly frightening is that unless modern medicine intervenes, many of us will wind up with similar memory loss, though from a different cause—Alzheimer's disease. When you're sixty-five, there's a one in ten chance you are affected by Alzheimer's. By the time you're over eighty-five, there's almost a one in two chance you have the disease, according to the Alzheimer's Association. Some medical researchers believe we would all get Alzheimer's if we lived long enough.

Alzheimer's is the most common cause of dementia among the 35 million Americans sixty-five and older (the greatest number of seniors in the nation's history). An estimated 4.5 million Americans have Alzheimer's, with 100,000 people a year dying of complications of the disease. As baby boomers age, that number will grow, and the number of Alzheimer's sufferers will grow with it—unless a medical breakthrough intervenes. At the current rate, the number of Alzheimer's cases is expected to almost triple by 2050, according to the National Institute on Aging.

Luckily for those of us who are under fifty, researchers gain a better understanding every year of how the brain works, how memories are formed, and how to stop the damaging plaques and tangles that form in the brains of Alzheimer's sufferers and that result in memory loss and dementia.

It isn't just Alzheimer's that makes people entering their golden years nervous. Even in healthy seniors, declining memory is a fact of life. Some neurons shrink with age in areas important to learning, memory, and other higher-level functions. As a result, as we get older, we may have more trouble remembering names, the location of car keys, or the location of the car itself. These "senior moments" can be both frustrating and frightening. Of course, part of the fear comes from the uncertainty about whether the forgetfulness is just a harmless mental slip or the first sign of Alzheimer's.

The prospect of memory loss is so unnerving because we are, in many ways, the sum of our memories. They define who we are. Memories tie us to our past, to our family and friends, and to the events that have shaped our lives—the weddings, births, deaths, successes, and failures along the way. Memories also instruct us, offering us lessons in the ways of the world. If we didn't remember, we wouldn't learn. The sum of our experiences—our memories—informs our worldview and sensibilities. You could say whatever wisdom we have is the product of our memories. In this way, they not only serve as a storehouse of information but also shape how we view the future. It should be no surprise, then, that the ability to hope and plan depends on memory.

REMEMBERING AND FORGETTING

What exactly is a memory? We tend to think our memories exist like some sort of neurological library or photo album. When we want to retrieve a memory of a specific event—a wedding or a birthday, for example—we retrieve the book or album that contains all the memories of that occasion. That is not the way memory works, though. The University of California professor James McGaugh, in many ways the father of memory research in the United States, told me our recollections are more like a net. When we want to call up the memory of an important event, we pull the various strands of the net. The images of the wedding come from one part of the brain, the smells from another, the sounds from another, the emotional memory from still another. The more strands or connections we have, the stronger the memory.

In a famous experiment that demonstrates this point, one group of test subjects was shown pictures of unfamiliar faces and the names that went with them. The second group was given the same faces and their occupations. In the experiment, the name and occupation given to each picture was the same. For example, one man was named Baker for one group and was a baker for the other group. Another was named Potter for one group and held a job as a potter for the other. When the separate groups were shown the faces later and asked to recall the name or the occupation, depending on the group, many more people remembered the occupation than the name. This is known as the Baker/baker experiment.

You may have had this experience yourself when you encountered a casual acquaintance you hadn't seen for a while. You can remember everything about that person—his job, the number of children he has, where you saw him last—but you do not remember his name. Why is that?

In the Baker/baker experiment, test subjects were much

more likely to remember a particular person was a baker rather than the name Baker because the job creates more connections in our brains. We are able to smell the bread baking, taste the bread, remember experiences we've had at bakeries. The name Baker does not create the same strong web of connections (unless, of course, we know someone else named Baker). It works the same way in the example of the casual acquaintance and in many aspects of our lives.

In fact, we filter out most of what we see every day. For the most part, these details don't even register. We can see something unremarkable every day and not even notice. You could think of our brains as acting more as filters allowing almost all the incoming information to pass unremembered, rather than as sponges soaking it up. If you don't believe me, think about the penny. You have no doubt seen a penny a thousand times. Probably more. Which way is Lincoln's head facing? What else is on the front of the penny? Does it say "Liberty"? How about "In God We Trust"? You don't remember because the penny is so ordinary. So unremarkable. So forgettable. This is just one of the thousands of details that wash over us every day of our lives. If we remembered everything—and there are some who do, with devastating consequences—we would be overwhelmed with details and would not be able to function in the world. We are experts at extracting the gist of an experience. This is how we learn. We may not remember what color shirt we were wearing or the day of the week, but we would likely retain a lifelong memory of getting stung by a bee as a child or the first time we rode a bike.

Our brains are constantly on the lookout for what is different—what is unusual—and emotional memories are stronger than unemotional ones. Memory is the act of storing information and then retrieving it when you need it. It sounds simple, but how many of us can say we've never forgotten where we parked the car at the mall or the airport? Usually, we weren't paying attention. The first step to remembering something is to make sure you are really noticing it.

A MEMORY "WORKOUT"

Scott Hagwood was the U.S. memory champion for four years running. He flew to Atlanta to teach me some of his mnemonic tricks. For example, he is constantly being quizzed on the names of the four or six or eight people he just met. With unflagging good cheer, Hagwood always gets the names right. Here's how he does it. When he is introduced to someone, he tries to think of someone else he knows with the same name and then one distinguishing physical characteristic about the person he just met. In that way, he is able to make the name something more than an abstraction. If he met someone named Baker, he would think of someone else he knew with the name. He would also pick out the cowlick or the crooked nose—some physical attribute that sets that person apart in order to add a visual memory. Hagwood's recall in situations like this is flawless, but he hasn't always had this ability.

Memory is something we need to work on, like a muscle, Hagwood says. Hagwood's story is a case in point. Hagwood did not do particularly well is school, nor was he born with a photographic memory. He graduated from the University of Tennessee, Knoxville with a degree in chemical engineering, but was by no means a standout. He struggled to remember things in college and left school feeling inadequate about his mental abilities. "I wasn't the sharpest tool in the shed," he likes to say.

At age thirty-six, Hagwood was diagnosed with thyroid cancer. He learned that one of the side effects of chemotherapy was memory loss. Hagwood decided to fight against that by working on his memory. Hagwood read books by Tony Buzan, a Briton who has written a number of books on improving memory, and he began "working out" with decks of playing cards. For hours every day, Hagwood worked on his memory.

Cured of cancer, Hagwood decided in 2001 to enter the USA Memory Championship, an Olympics of the mind in which contestants are asked to remember impossibly long strings of numbers, names, faces, a poem, and other mnemonic challenges. Hagwood won, and he kept on winning. In fact, he won all four years he entered the USA Memory Championship. Hagwood now has a book of his own, *Memory Power: You Can Develop a Great Memory—America's Grand Master Shows You How*.

I spent an hour with Hagwood for a documentary I did on memory. He gave me a quick explanation of the memory trick he and other top memory "athletes" use. Their technique involves converting names, numbers, cards, or whatever else they want to remember into moving images—experiences—that they place in their minds around their virtual homes or some other well-known place. The theory is that we are much more likely to remember a moving picture than the name of a card. For example, the four of hearts, to Hagwood, is a rabbit.

"I can feel the fur, and I can see the whiskers moving," Hagwood told me. "Our physical eye is trained for movement. So is the mental eye." Creating a mental picture of a rabbit creates many more connections in the brain than trying to remember "four of hearts" or even an image of the card. Research shows emotional memories are stronger than unemotional ones, and a rabbit certainly conjures up more emotion than a playing card.

If the four of hearts was the first card in a deck Hagwood was memorizing, he would place the rabbit, in his mind's eye, in one corner of his living room. The next card he would place in the next corner. That way he can work his way around his house in his mind and never skip a card. He can also work backwards simply by reversing the order in which he makes his way through his house.

Hagwood can memorize an entire deck of cards in under three minutes and nine decks of cards, in order, in less than an hour. He can memorize a sequence of more than eight hundred numbers in an hour. To see Hagwood in action memorizing cards is to be amazed. I went through half a deck of cards, rapid fire, and he proceeded to list them back for me. He then put me through the paces, and in the space of about ten minutes, I was able to memorize ten cards. A modest accomplishment, but I find myself still using his memory techniques. The mind is like a muscle, Hagwood told me repeatedly. You should exercise your brain the way you would exercise your body. Hagwood insists his gifts are available to anyone who wants to hit the mental gym.

Interestingly, Hagwood says he forgets many of the mundane details of his life, just like the rest of us. He puts his car keys in the same drawer in his house every day so he doesn't lose them. Hagwood jokes that when his wife is asked what it's like to live with someone with a perfect memory, she answers, "I wouldn't know."

Incidentally, if you want to remember where you parked your car in a large parking lot, see where you are and make a mental picture. If you are parked in section 5B, you might create a mental picture of a giant hand sticking out of your car with a oversized bee on each finger. The more outlandish the image, the more likely you are to remember it.

PROTECTING THE MIND

Having the ability to remember names or other facts is one thing, but keeping our minds sharp and preserving our memories is much more basic to who we are and to living well in our senior years. What can we do to keep our brains sharp? After all, what good is a healthy body unless we are mentally "there" to enjoy it? Are we genetically predestined to succeed or fail mentally in old age? What, if anything, can we do on our own to protect our brains from the ravages of Alzheimer's?

Alzheimer's is named for Alois Alzheimer, a German physician who was dedicated to the study of the brain. He gave a lecture to the South-West German Society of Alienists in

November 1906 that forever linked his name with the disease. At the meeting of alienists—an antiquated term for psychiatrists who are expert in the legal aspects of mental illness—Alzheimer described *eine eigenartige Erkrankung der Hirnrinde*, an unusual disease of the cerebral cortex in a mental patient who had died and whose brain had been sent to him. The patient, Frau Auguste D., died in her fifties at a Munich mental asylum after suffering from memory loss, disorientation, trouble reading and writing, and hallucinations. Alzheimer noticed that her cerebral cortex appeared to be thinner than normal. He also described what have become the hallmarks of the disease that took his name: the buildup of beta-amyloid plaques in the spaces between the brain's nerve cells and the neurofibrillary tangles inside the nerve cells. A year later, Alzheimer's second case entered a university psychiatric clinic in Munich, a demented fifty-six-year-old named Johann F.

Most people get some plaque in their brains as they get older, but in Alzheimer's disease, the beta-amyloid plaques develop first in areas of the brain used for memory and other cognitive functions. Illustrations of these plaques generally depict them looking something like dust balls between the brain cells. Many researchers now believe the buildup of plaques between cells is a last-ditch effort by the brain to keep harmful beta-amyloid away from neurons. Increasingly, scientists think the plaques themselves do not cause harm, and that the real culprit may be something called oligomers. These are small, discrete clumps of a handful to a dozen or so beta-amyloid proteins. Researchers at Northwestern University suggest that these, not the plaques, may be the real vandals in the brain, attaching to a critical location on nerve synapses in the brain and disrupting communication between neurons. Unable to communicate, the neurons eventually die. When enough of these neurons die, our mental abilities dim.

The neurofibrillary tangles Alzheimer saw in the brain of Frau Auguste are twisted protein threads inside nerve cells. These don't exist in healthy individuals. The bulk of these tangles are made up of the protein tau, which builds up in patients with Alzheimer's disease after being pulled away from structures inside neurons. The end result of all this may be miscommunication between cells and, later, cell death.

A third physiological feature of Alzheimer's—not noticed by Alzheimer himself—is the slow loss of connections between neurons. Eventually, they can't function properly, and they die. As neurons die across areas of the brain, those regions atrophy—like the muscles of someone who is unable to move.

Genetic factors determine an estimated 40 to 80 percent of our cognitive abilities and also affect our risk of getting Alzheimer's disease. In 1992, researchers found that certain forms of the apolipoprotein E gene, commonly referred to as the *APOE* gene, influences our risk of Alzheimer's. The *APOE* ϵ*4* gene appears to increase our risk. It is found in 40 percent of people with Alzheimer's, although there are many people with the gene who never develop the disease. Conversely, 60 percent of people with Alzheimer's do not have the gene. The rarely occurring *APOE* ϵ*2* gene may provide some protection against Alzheimer's, while the *APOE* ϵ*3* gene appears to be neutral.

The FDA has approved a handful of drugs to treat Alzheimer's. They do not work for everyone. Even in those people the drugs help, they do not stop the progression of the disease and are only mildly effective at slowing it for a period of months to a few years. But every year, scientists are making great strides in understanding both Alzheimer's and how memories are formed, and they have developed compounds that radically improve the memories of fruit flies and mice. Pharmaceutical companies are now working hard, building on these breakthroughs to extend the results to humans.

Dozens of clinical trials are under way, testing the safety and efficacy of dozens of compounds designed to treat Alzheimer's and mild cognitive impairment. Cholesterol-lowering statins are one class of drugs under investigation. They have shown some promise in clinical trials at slowing the progression of Alzheimer's disease. The results are mixed, and doctors are cautioning against recommending statins to treat Alzheimer's until more data is in. That data is on the way.

At this writing, two large, multicenter trials have begun, testing the effectiveness of two different statins in the prevention of Alzheimer's. Another found a link between nonsteroidal anti-inflammatory drugs, like ibuprofen, and a lower risk of Alzheimer's. Raloxifene (Evista), a drug used to promote bone growth in postmenopausal women, has also been associated with a lower risk of Alzheimer's. Women taking the osteoporosis drug had a 33 percent lower risk of developing mild cognitive impairment, often a precursor to Alzheimer's, compared to the placebo group. Still, it's far too early to be taking any of these for the sole purpose of avoiding Alzheimer's.

Alzheimer's Vaccine?

In the future, we may be able to get immunized against Alzheimer's. Nothing exists yet, but tests in which antibodies were injected into the brains of genetically engineered mice have succeeded in reducing amyloid deposits and reversing the development of neurofibrillary tangles.

The ultimate goal of all this research, of course, is nothing less than preventing or dramatically slowing Alzheimer's, something science has thus far been unable to do. That means, for the time being anyway, it is up to us to do what we can to live in a way that lessens our chances of ever getting Alzheimer's. If you have a family history of the disease, you need to be particularly mindful of behaviors that add to your risk and do what you can to lead a lifestyle that may actually reduce your chances of getting the disease.

HOLD THAT THOUGHT

Beginning in childhood, the way in which we live influences whether we are putting ourselves at greater or lesser risk for Alzheimer's. Even delaying the onset of Alzheimer's through healthy living is a worthwhile goal. Another year or two without the disease is another year or two of living life to the fullest. Remember our goal: to maximize our life span and remain mentally and physically fit for as long as possible. Incidentally, Alzheimer's not only profoundly affects our quality of life, it is also associated with a dramatically reduced life span. If you are seventy years old and get Alzheimer's, you can expect to live 8 more years if you are a woman and about 4.5 more years if you are a man. That's half of what a woman that age without Alzheimer's could expect to live and about a third of what a man that age could expect to live.

Dr. Gary Small is a professor of aging at the University of California, Los Angeles medical school, director of UCLA's Memory and Aging Research Center, and the author of several books on keeping the brain healthy and our memories strong. Small, among others, argues that mental health and physical health are linked. In other words, a healthy body, to a large degree, means a healthy brain. Small advocates exercising, reducing stress through meditation and other means, performing stimulating mental activities, and eating a healthy diet. He recommends a Mediterranean diet, with fish, olive oil, nuts, vegetables, and fresh fruits, which together lower the risk for heart disease and Alzheimer's.

"Eating fish once a week or just walking ten minutes a day. We looked at it over the next five years, and if everybody did that, and if our assumptions were true, we would reduce the number of cases in the United States by a million in just five years," Small told me in an interview.

Cold-water fish, such as salmon, halibut, mackerel, sardines, and herring, all contain the omega-3 fatty acid docosahexaenoic acid (DHA). DHA is involved in a number of brain processes, including many related to nerve cell communication. Scientists believe DHA helps protect the brain against the cell damage caused by Alzheimer's disease. In mice, DHA appeared to protect against beta-amyloid production, accumulation, and toxicity.

Because fish high in DHA can also contain mercury, dioxin, polychlorinated biphenyls (PCBs), and other harmful metals, eating them more than once a week can be dangerous. Another alternative is to take an omega-3 supplement made from algae. A third option is to eat eggs produced by chickens consuming DHA-rich feed, such as flaxseed. DHA-enriched eggs are more expensive than standard eggs but taste the same and offer an alternative source of omega-3 fatty acid.

Fruits and vegetables also appear to help. One study following more than thirteen thousand older women for more than a decade found those who ate the most green, leafy vegetables experienced slower cognitive decline than those who ate the fewest. Vitamins C and E and beta-carotene, found in carrots and other fruits and vegetables, may protect against cognitive decline, while deficiencies in vitamin B_{12} and folic acid may increase the risk. A note of caution: like fish, too much vitamin E can be dangerous.

Light to moderate alcohol use may reduce the risk of Alzheimer's, while heavy alcohol use increases the risk.

Researchers are looking into whether the main chemical compound in the spice turmeric, which makes curry yellow, may be a valuable dietary tool for warding off Alzheimer's. Turmeric has been used for thousands of years as an anti-inflammatory, and inflammation in the brain occurs during the neurodegenerative process that accompanies Alzheimer's. So it would make sense that a substance with anti-inflammatory properties might help. A study with mice suggests the yellow pigment in turmeric, called curcumin, can suppress amyloid accumulation, which contributes to Alzheimer's. Clinical trials in humans are under way. Because turmeric has been used in food for so long (it was around when Marco Polo visited Asia in the thirteenth century), side effects are less of a concern than they are in drug trials of compounds that are concocted in the lab. Researchers began looking into curcumin when they noticed that Indians experienced low rates of Alzheimer's, heart disease, and several cancers. These low rates went away when Indians moved to western countries and abandoned their traditional diets. This suggested the Indians' protection against these ailments was not genetic.

Much has been made of the brain-boosting powers of *Ginkgo biloba*, but there is little evidence the much-touted supplement does much to either improve our mental abilities or to ward off Alzheimer's.

Aside from eating healthy foods, there appear to be a number of foods to avoid if we want to keep our brains healthy. They include trans-fatty acids, which are found in fried foods, processed baked goods, and some margarines; saturated fats, which are found in meat and full-fat dairy products; artificial sweeteners; and sugar. Cigarette smoking also heightens the risk for dementia.

Advice from the Experts

The Alzheimer's Association of America recommends reducing the risk factors for dementia by treating depression and controlling hypertension, diabetes, and heart disease by quitting smoking, controlling blood pressure, lowering cholesterol, and avoiding obesity.

A diet containing a lot of fat, especially saturated and trans fats, has been linked to Alzheimer's disease and other cognitive loss among the elderly. If you add a lot of copper to a high-fat diet, the Alzheimer's risk skyrockets.

One study that followed Chicagoans sixty-five and older found a high-fat, high-copper diet resulted in the equivalent of nineteen years of mental aging in just six years, based on cognitive tests. Interestingly, those who ate a high-copper diet without a lot of fat did not show a higher than average mental decline during the course of the study.

In case you're wondering, such organ meats as liver and shellfish are foods with the highest levels of copper. Other foods high in copper include nuts, seeds, legumes, whole grains, chocolate, and some fruits. The recommended daily allowance for copper is 0.9 milligrams. A single ounce of liver contains 4 milligrams of copper; a lobster tail contains 2.3 milligrams. If you eat 6 ounces of roasted peanuts, you would be right at the 0.9-milligram daily allowance.

* * *

If you want to adopt a lifestyle that lowers your risk of developing Alzheimer's and dementia, exercise. Older adults who exercised at least three times a week were much less likely to develop dementia than those who were less active, according to a recent study published in the *Archives of Internal Medicine*. The types of exercise that appeared to help were walking, hiking, bicycling, aerobics, and weight training. The study did not show that exercise prevented dementia, but that those who exercised developed dementia a third less often. On the flip side, poor physical function may be associated with an increased risk of dementia and Alzheimer's.

Leisure activities also appear to play a role in reducing the risk of Alzheimer's, possibly because they are a source of ongoing intellectual and social stimulation. Remember the Okinawans? Alzheimer's is far less common among elderly Okinawans, who engage in such leisure activities as gardening and tend to have strong social networks that keep them engaged with family and neighbors into very old age.

A longer education also is associated with better mental functioning in middle age and beyond. College graduates are less likely to get Alzheimer's than high school graduates.

Also, people in jobs that are more mentally demanding appear less likely to get Alzheimer's. Jobs were assessed on criteria such as the complexity of work with data, people, and things. Complexity of work with data considers whether the job involves mentally taxing activities, such as computing and analyzing. Complexity of work with people takes into consideration whether the job involves negotiating, supervising, or other challenging work relationships. Complexity of work with things looks at whether the job involves manipulating objects, operating machinery, or other precision work.

Ross Andel did research with James Mortimer at the University of South Florida in Tampa, using data from the Swedish Twin Registry. Among the more than ten thousand twins registered in the ongoing Swedish study, Andel and Mortimer found twenty-two same-sex pairs with occupations that differed with respect to complexity of work, and one of the twins developed some form of dementia. In twenty-one of those cases, the demented twin had the less-complicated job. For those engaged in complex work requiring people skills, the future risk of dementia seems to be relatively small, Andel says.

There are life circumstances that place you at greater risk of getting Alzheimer's, most of them apparently because of the additional stress involved. If you have never been married, grew up in a single-parent home, or were born after three or more siblings, you are at greater risk for Alzheimer's. Sustaining physical or emotional abuse during childhood or your teenage years or losing a parent also tip the odds against you.

In a French study, elderly people who were married had a significantly lower rate of Alzheimer's disease in their mideighties and beyond than did those who were widowed, divorced, or never married. Growing up in the suburbs, as opposed to the city, also is associated with a lower risk for Alzheimer's disease.

Scientists' search for biochemical links to Alzheimer's has looked at a number of possibilities. Research has found a high level of the amino acid homocysteine is associated with a greater risk for developing Alzheimer's. Homocysteine has also been linked to heart disease. Levels of the amino acid can be reduced with folic acid and vitamins B_6 and B_{12}. There are also associations between Alzheimer's and risk factors for stroke, such as high blood pressure, that begin in midlife. Researchers are also studying a potential link between Alzheimer's and diabetes. Diabetes is associated with a greater incidence of several forms of dementia, including Alzheimer's. One study of a large group of older priests, nuns, and brothers found that diabetics were 65 percent more likely to have Alzheimer's. There is also a biochemical connection. In Alzheimer's, an amyloid protein builds up in the brain. In type 2 diabetes, a different amyloid protein builds up—in the pancreas.

EXERCISE YOUR MIND

In addition to diet and exercise, the latest research suggests there is something else we can do to improve our odds of at least significantly delaying the onset of the dreaded disease. We can exercise our minds. This probably doesn't come as a surprise, we are all familiar with the phrase "use it or lose it."

Small serves as medical director for a private company called the Memory Fitness Institute, which is launching "brain boot camps" to help stimulate the minds of people in their golden years. In addition to exercising, improving diet, and reducing stress, participants engage in word games and other mental exercises. For example, they write with their opposite hand or practice remembering a list of words by creating zany stories to link them together.

In what amounted to a test run of the two-week brain boot camp, Small and his colleagues at UCLA took positron-emission tomography (PET) scans measuring blood flow in the brains of seventeen individuals. At the end of the fourteen days, the researchers took another brain scan. They found less brain metabolism in the region of the brain linked to memory and other cognitive functions. Small told me in an interview that this showed how these test subjects were able to use their brains more efficiently in just two weeks. The individuals also reported having better memory and performed better on a test. Admittedly, this is a very small study over a very short amount of time, but large-scale, population-based studies show time and again that education and mentally stimulating lives appear to protect us from age-related mental decline.

Even when the characteristic plaques and tangles in the brain that comprise Alzheimer's are present, education appears to help fight against their effects. More educated people are able to live longer without showing symptoms of Alzheimer's. They also show fewer symptoms than others with the same number of plaques and tangles in the brain. That means the symptoms will not appear until the disease is physiologically far more advanced than it is in those with less education. The more educated brains are somehow able to compensate for the damage, possibly because the initial connections in the brain are stronger or because their brains have adopted alternative pathways that avoid the damaged areas.

Autopsies back up these clinical observations. Researchers at Rush University Medical Center Alzheimer's Disease Center in Chicago, in an ongoing study of aging among members of forty religious communities, found people with more formal education were able to sustain a greater buildup of plaques in the brain tissue.

PET scan studies have found the same thing. Damage from Alzheimer's reduces the flow of blood in the brain. The more serious the Alzheimer's damage in the brain, the lower the blood flow. You would expect the symptoms to follow suit, and they do in many Alzheimer's sufferers. But in well-educated patients, that doesn't happen. If you are well educated or had a high IQ before you were diagnosed, or if you had a mentally challenging job, then your symptoms would be much less severe than those in a person with the same blood flow minus the education, IQ, or job. Life activities such as reading, traveling, going for walks, gardening, and playing cards also seem to help give you the kind of brain that can better deal with Alzheimer's.

This ability has prompted researchers to come up with the theory of cognitive reserve. A person with cognitive reserve essentially has extra capacity, which would have to be used up before symptoms started appearing. Someone with cognitive reserve would be able to tolerate more brain damage before showing a decline in mental functioning because his or her brain networks are either more efficient or more flexible (or both) than those in a less-educated person who does not have cognitive reserve. Not everyone agrees with this theory, but proponents point to mounting evidence that those who have used their brains more throughout their lives are better protected.

Evidence suggests almost any type of mental or social activity is beneficial, and the more you do, the better. Researchers have yet to figure out if one particular mental activity is superior to the rest in terms of warding off the symptoms of Alzheimer's or compensating for the brain damage associated with the disease.

If the Alzheimer's research wasn't enough to get you to break out the Scrabble game, consider this: Cognitive reserve seems to do more than ward off Alzheimer's. It also appears to help patients who have suffered from traumatic brain injuries. Shelli R. Kesler, a senior research scientist at Stanford University's Center for Interdisciplinary Brain Sciences Research, has looked at magnetic resonance imaging (MRI) scans of twenty-five patients with traumatic brain injuries. Kesler and colleagues at Stanford and Brigham Young University found that brain size and education were good predictors of postinjury IQ, regardless of the severity of the injury. That suggests more education means less vulnerability to brain injury.

Kesler says more education means more neuroplasticity. Neuroplasticity is the brain's ability to change. Neuroplasticity is stronger when we are younger. Anyone who has seen how quickly a child can master a foreign language knows that. But Kesler says neuroplasticity never ends. You can, in fact, teach an old dog new tricks. It just might take a little longer.

If you are an "old dog" reading this, you should be trying to learn new tricks on a continuing basis. Challenge your mind. Pick up an instrument. Learn a language. Read books. Do word games or math puzzles. Learning actually changes the shape, size, and number of neurons in our brains. The more you learn, the more protection your brain appears to have against damage later on.

"You can always learn," Kesler says. "The more you learn, the bigger reserve you are going to have." That's the good news. The bad news is we need to keep challenging ourselves in different ways, she says. Don't do the same type of mental exercise every day. Do a variety of challenging verbal and visual-spatial exercises. If you have mastered the crossword puzzle in your local newspaper, try sudoku. As you master one level of difficulty, go to the next level.

"Challenge yourself. Move up and progress to the harder ones," she advises. "When you're getting good at one thing, you want to do something you're not very good at."

It comes back to the analogy the memory champion Scott Hagwood likes to make: exercising the brain is like exercising the body. If you went to the gym, you would not use only the bench press every day, nor would you use the same amount of weight every day. You would use different machines and, if you were really working at it, you would probably start lifting heavier weights. You want to build strength in your brain in the same way. Make sure you are exercising your brain every day—in new and challenging ways. Chasing life is as much about keeping your mind sharp and functional as it is your body. Getting older doesn't mean you have to forget your past or your present.

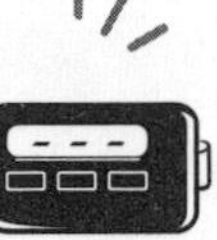

Paging Dr. Gupta

- ✓ Exercise your brain in different ways. Find problems that you have difficulty solving. The more you challenge your mind the better.
- ✓ Exercise your body; it helps your brain.
- ✓ Stay social and enjoy spirited discussions.
- ✓ Even if you're an old dog, learn a new trick—the more you learn, the more you protect your mind.
- ✓ Make sure you get enough "brain food," including fish oil, vitamins E and B, and folic acid.
- ✓ Add the spice turmeric to your diet—it may ward off Alzheimer's.

CHAPTER 6

Taming the Beast

President Richard Nixon declared war on cancer in his State of the Union address in 1971. Nixon wanted U.S. researchers to tackle the vexing problem with the same intensity as the Manhattan Project during World War II and the race to the Moon in the 1960s. Congress followed the president's lead and passed the National Cancer Act, which called for the defeat of cancer by the time the nation celebrated its bicentennial, in 1976.

As anybody who has ever been touched by cancer knows, the sometimes ruthless disease was not eradicated by the bicentennial, nor does its extinction appear imminent. Despite the millions of dollars that continue to be poured into research, despite the brilliant minds that have tackled the problem, despite the dedication of researchers around the world, modern medicine has not conquered the "Big C." They have not found the switch to turn off cells that are dividing out of control.

Cancer remains widespread, striking 1.2 million Americans

a year and killing more than 500,000. That's about 1,500 people a day, dead of cancer. And the incidence of several cancers is rising, according to the National Cancer Institute. They include breast cancer in women; prostate and testicular cancer in men; skin melanoma, and cancers of the thyroid, kidney, and esophagus.

Even though cancer remains a killer, it would be wrong to say cancer researchers have come up empty-handed. They have not. Medical research has turned up many ingenious ways to tame what cancer patients call "the beast." They have developed major advances in the treatment of a wide range of cancers. The total cancer mortality rate started to decline in 1990 and has been falling about 1 percent a year. Some cancers are now treated more like chronic illnesses, and many childhood cancers that were once fatal are now curable. For example, the cure rate for testicular cancer in young men was 5 percent when President Nixon declared his war on cancer. It's now 80 percent. For all cancers, the five-year survival rates have risen from 50 percent when President Nixon was in office to more than 65 percent. Death rates are declining for the four most common cancers: prostate, breast, lung, and colorectal.

There are now more than 10 million cancer survivors in the United States. That means more than one in thirty Americans has "tamed the beast," which is a remarkable number. Even so, progress has been maddeningly slow.

These are dry facts, statistics that do not do justice to the very real, very human trauma and turmoil a diagnosis of cancer brings not only for patients but their families.

NO LONGER A DEATH SENTENCE

As a neurosurgeon, I see one of the most virulent cancers, glioblastoma, a particularly malignant brain tumor that afflicts seven thousand Americans a year. The five-year survival rate for a glioblastoma patient is 3 percent. Brain surgery is just the first step for these patients. Radiation therapy and chemotherapy often follow. From the moment they hear the diagnosis, the perspective of these cancer patients—and their families—telescopes. Instead of planning for retirement or making other long-term plans, they focus on what they want to do this year, what they want to do now. Cancer often brings out remarkable courage in people. Sometimes, it brings lives into sharp focus. I've even heard survivors say getting cancer was a blessing in disguise because it caused them to realign their priorities to bring more meaning and joy into their lives. Of course, no one would choose cancer. The treatment regimen for cancer patients is demanding, and the outcome is by no means guaranteed.

In 2005, I spent time at one of the leading cancer hospitals in the country, M.D. Anderson in Houston, Texas, for an award-winning documentary on cancer titled *Taming the Beast*. M.D. Anderson conducts more clinical trials than any other facility in the country. You don't have to be there long to realize how egalitarian cancer is. Cancer strikes rich and poor, black and white, women, men, and children. No one is immune. Not even doctors.

Dr. Samuel Hassenbusch III is a neurosurgeon at M.D. Anderson and is world renowned for his chronic pain treatments.

In addition to an MD, he has a PhD and has published more than one hundred articles in scientific journals. At this writing, he is president-elect of the Texas Association of Neurological Surgeons. The fifty-one-year-old Texan, who wears cowboy boots and rides a motorcycle, is used to being very much in control of his life. But in May 2005, the doctor's life took an unfamiliar path. He began losing control. It started with headaches. His right temple would throb. He would take an acetaminophen, and his headache would feel better for a while. Then, the headache would return. At first, he suspected an ear problem. Perhaps he was grinding his teeth at night. Then he started worrying. The cancer doctor began worrying he himself might have cancer. He dismissed his anxiety as the product of an active imagination, the result of being around cancer patients all day. So Hassenbusch took control. To prove to himself he was being a hypochondriac, he went to a head and neck doctor and had an MRI done at another hospital. For some reason, one of the films of his MRI was left up on the light box. He was one of the first to see it. What he saw was his worst nightmare.

"I could see it clear as day. It was a classic glioblastoma," Hassenbusch recalls. Then he checked out the name on the film. His name. He couldn't believe it. What are the chances the neurosurgeon who operates on glioblastomas has one himself? If this was a made-for-TV movie, the critics would pan it as unbelievable. Hassenbusch actually thought he was dreaming—and he wanted to wake up.

"When I saw that, I kept rubbing my eyes and pinching myself. It was like one of those weird dreams. It was surreal," Hassenbusch says. Unfortunately, it was all too real. Samuel Hassenbusch III, MD, PhD, went from being a doctor to being a patient in a split second. Not only that, he went from being a brain surgeon who operated on people with glioblastomas to someone with a glioblastoma in need of surgery.

There is nothing you can do to prepare yourself for the knowledge you have cancer, especially a virulent one like a glioblastoma. Even though he was a doctor who was around cancer patients all day, Hassenbusch was stunned. The doctor who had not taken a sick day since eighth grade now had to prepare himself for surgery and an uncertain future.

"I saw the next year of my life flash before my eyes," he recalls. "I do this for a living." Hassenbusch had performed surgery on glioblastoma patients thirty times. He knew the risks and the slim chance that the surgery would get the entire tumor. The hardest part of the diagnosis was telling his friends, Hassenbusch says now.

"It was a tremendous shock," he says. "Interestingly, what you see in their eyes is, 'What would I do?' All you can do is pick the cards up and play the cards the best we can." As is the case with many patients, cancer also made Hassenbusch turn to God, a renewed spirituality he says helped him in the difficult months that followed.

Knowing he would be asked after the operation for his name, the date, and the president, Hassenbusch put up Post-it Notes all over his house. He wanted to regain control. He also picked the date and time of his surgery, the surgeons, the scrub nurse, the circulating nurse, and the anesthesiologist. The surgeons performed a temporal lobectomy. Fortunately for Hassenbusch, the tumor was nondominant and anterior. In the world of neurosurgery, that was at least some good news. While these tumors and their removal can dramatically affect speech and vision, Hassenbusch's tumor's location made it less likely for that to happen. Still, a glioblastoma is gray in color, making it hard to distinguish from the rest of the normal brain. It also often has these rubbery tentacles that invade and destroy brain tissue all around it. They are the most difficult tumors to remove in their entirety. He sailed through the operation, and four days later, he even went back to work to attend a meeting. A week later, he performed surgery with a colleague on a pain patient.

After his operation, Hassenbusch started both vaccine therapy and chemotherapy and went back to work half time. He says his experience has taught him to be more empathetic toward his patients. Even before his diagnosis, Hassenbusch says he was "old school," taking the time to listen to his patients. Now, he says he works hard to give them results as soon as possible after tests are performed and to make the scheduling as convenient as possible. And, he says, he really tries to listen to his patients and what they are going through. As a doctor, the talk is about medicine and treatments, Hassenbusch says. As a patient, it is more about attitude and setting goals.

He still receives chemotherapy and vaccine therapy every month and will continue to do so at least until he hits the twenty-four-month mark. He recently had an MRI, and there was no sign of tumor. Nothing even suspicious. He also ran in a 5K road race to raise money for cancer research and was the lead motorcycle in a six-hundred-motorcycle rally, the grand marshal in another fund-raiser. His headaches had started almost exactly a year earlier, just after the same road race. His goal after surgery was to get better enough to run the race again.

"All things considered, I've had a great year," Hassenbusch says. Thirty-five years after President Nixon declared war on cancer, Hassenbusch thinks the tide is turning in favor of medicine.

"We're beginning to win the war," he says. "It's been a long war. A hard war."

All the hard work unraveling genes and chromosomes is starting to pay off, Hassenbusch says. Before his diagnosis, he gave a talk in Washington to congressional staffers involved with health-care issues. For the talk, he prepared a list of all the various enzymes now known to be in some way involved in cancer formation and growth, the product of years of research by hundreds of labs and thousands of researchers around the world. It was an enormous list. All that painstaking, often frustrating research has produced a body of knowledge capable of tracing the chemical pathways for many cancers. More than simply offering doctors a greater understanding of cancers, this increased knowledge gives doctors new and better tools to fight cancers.

NEW TREATMENTS

For many cancers, doctors can now use targeted molecular therapies instead of or in combination with chemotherapy. Targeted molecular therapy attacks the chemical pathway unique to the cancer, interrupting the cancer's ability to divide and grow. Targeted molecular therapies are "smart bombs" that stop the cancer's spread with minimal collateral damage to the surrounding cells. Traditional chemotherapy is less discriminate. It destroys rapidly dividing cells—cancer cells—but can also damage other cells elsewhere, such as the intestinal lining and bone marrow.

A lymphoma-fighting drug called rituximab (Rituxan) was the first targeted molecular therapy to hit the market, in 1997. Others have followed for breast cancer, colon cancer, and others. A number of potential targeted molecular therapies are in clinical trials for many more cancers.

"These are home run hits," Hassenbusch says, although a targeted therapy is not yet available for glioblastoma.

Quality of life has improved for most cancer patients, but for some the quantity of life after a cancer diagnosis remains about the same as it was when President Nixon declared war on the disease.

We cannot eliminate any chance of getting cancer, and as we get older, the odds of getting cancer increase. There are steps we can take to minimize our risks, though.

AVOIDING RISKS

Recent estimates from the Harvard School of Public Health and other institutions say nine controllable risk factors are responsible for a third of cancer deaths worldwide. Smokers and drinkers put themselves at the greatest cancer risk, according to the research, which was published in *The Lancet*, a well-respected British medical journal. The other cancer risk factors are obesity, inactivity, a diet with too few fruits and vegetables, unsafe sex, urban air pollution, indoor smoke from household fuels, and contaminated injections in health-care settings.

These are the greatest risk factors worldwide. We are fortunate in the United States that smoke from indoor cooking fires and contaminated injections are extremely rare. Also, cervical cancer screening through Pap tests here significantly lowers the cancer risk from unsafe sex, which is spread by the human papillomavirus (HPV), the virus responsible for nearly all cases of cervical cancer. In the developed world, however, we are guilty of obesity, inactivity, a diet lacking in fruits and vegetables, drinking alcohol, and smoking.

A 2006 study on cancer risks and prevention conducted by the American Cancer Society concluded that lifestyle changes could prevent as many as half of all cancer deaths in the United States. Think about it. Half of all cancer deaths. That's more than 250,000 people a year. That is not to say that people who get cancer are at fault. I do not want to blame cancer victims. But if you could lower your risk of cancer, why wouldn't you?

Nine Controllable Cancer Risks

1. Smoking
2. Alcohol
3. Obesity
4. Inactivity
5. A diet with too few fruits and vegetables
6. Unsafe sex
7. Urban air pollution
8. Indoor smoke from household fuels
9. Contaminated injections in health-care settings

At the top of the list of lifestyle choices that significantly raise the risk of cancer death is smoking. Cigarette smoke contains more than sixty carcinogens, and more than 170,000 cancer deaths in 2006 were caused by tobacco use, according to American Cancer Society estimates. Smoking cigarettes raises the risk for many types of cancer and accounts for about a third of all cancer deaths. In addition to lung cancer, cigarette smoking is also linked to cancer of the mouth, esophagus, stomach, pancreas, and bladder, among others.

Despite the common knowledge that cigarette smoking

can cause cancer, one in five adults smokes. Even so, continued public service campaigns, higher taxes, and other efforts have caused tobacco use to decline in the United States. Per capita cigarette consumption is now at its lowest level since the beginning of World War II. In case you were wondering, Kentucky, a big tobacco-growing state, has the highest percentage of adult smokers, 27.6 percent; Utah has the lowest, 10.5 percent.

If you do smoke, I don't want you to toss this book away and despair. Quitting now will eliminate most of the risk caused by smoking. In fact, smokers who quit can expect to live significantly longer than those who keep smoking. How much longer? One study found if you quit smoking at age thirty, you can expect to live ten years longer than if you continued smoking. Even quitting at age sixty adds three years of life expectancy, the study found.

No question, cigarettes are horribly addictive, but there are a number of effective treatments available for smokers who want to quit, and studies show most smokers do. Among them are nicotine patches, gum and other nicotine-replacement products, counseling, behavioral therapies, and medication. Some insurance plans cover smoking cessation treatments and, at this writing, forty-four states operate telephone counseling services for people who want to quit. Efforts to quit are generally most effective when several of these techniques are used simultaneously.

If you have any doubt at all about whether you should quit, think about increasing your chances of avoiding the pain and trauma of cancer. If that doesn't do the trick, consider the possibility of spending extra years with family and loved ones.

For nonsmokers, secondhand smoke poses a cancer risk, especially for people who live with smokers. Breathing secondhand cigarette smoke poses the same risks as smoking, though at lower levels. Overall, exposure to secondhand smoke has been decreasing for years, thanks to widening bans on smoking in public places. Even so, if you want to reduce your risk of cancer, avoid secondhand smoke.

FACTS AND MYTHS

Many of the products we use or consume every day have been implicated as potential cancer risks, from Teflon to beef, from cell phones to artificial sweeteners, from plastics to hormones in milk. Let's take a moment to separate the myth from the reality, remembering that little in science is certain—especially when you're trying to figure out what effect environmental factors have in our complex lives.

Bovine Growth Hormone

Most dairy cows in the United States receive injections of synthetic bovine growth hormone (BGH) to increase milk production. Dairy producers, the FDA, and Monsanto, the company that makes the growth hormone, say the hormone injections do not pose any health risk. Critics say BGH, also called bovine somatotropin (BST), could raise the risk of hormone-related cancers or lead to higher levels of insulinlike growth factor (IGF-1), which have been linked to cancers of the colon, breast, and prostate. Cancer fears have contributed to an increase in consumption of organic milk, which is considerably more expensive.

Although there is something inherently unsettling about drinking milk from cows injected with artificial growth hormone, the fears about BGH appear to be largely unfounded. The FDA asked Monsanto to test whether BGH is digested or absorbed, which would make it more dangerous. The findings: Rats fed large doses of BGH for twenty-eight days did not show any signs they were absorbing the hormone. And even though the slightly higher levels of IGF-1 in BGH-treated cows appears to translate into slightly higher levels of IGF-1 in the people drinking it, the change is small compared with the amount our bodies naturally produce. According to one estimate, we'd have to drink 95 quarts of milk to equal the amount of IGF-1 our bodies produce every day in our salvia and digestive tract. The long-term risk of not getting enough calcium in our diet almost certainly outweighs the additional risks posed by dairy herds treated with BGH.

At first blush, BGH's link to cancer appears to fall squarely in the myth category. But regulators in the European Union (EU) are not as comfortable with BGH as their U.S. counterparts. The EU prohibits the use of BGH in beef cattle or dairy cows for nontherapeutic reasons. The EU also bans the importation of American beef raised on growth hormones, which speeds the time between birth and slaughter. (Grass-fed beef, though more expensive, is likely to be lower in fat and contain higher levels of healthy omega-3 fatty acids and conjugated linoleic acid, which animal studies show may lower the risk of cancer.)

While I'm on the subject of the EU, European regulators require foods from genetically modified crops to be labeled as such. So do Japan, China, Australia, and New Zealand. There is a pervasive fear of these genetically modified organisms (GMOs), which are bioengineered by adding genes from other plants or organisms to make them resistant to pests or spoiling, improve their flavor, or give them some other beneficial characteristic. Despite the alarm caused by "frankenfoods," the American Cancer Society says there is no evidence GMOs increase or decrease the risk of cancer. Of course, GMOs are relatively new, so no long-term studies have been done.

On the flip side, there is no evidence yet that organic food, grown free of pesticides or genetic modification, reduces cancer risk. In fact, the American Cancer Society does not see the low levels of herbicides and pesticides sometimes remaining on the fruits and vegetables we eat as a cancer threat. There is a greater risk from not eating enough fruits and vegetables, according to the nonprofit organization.

Meats, Packaged or Cooked

Most lunch meats, bacon, ham, sausage, and hot dogs contain sodium nitrite, a preservative used primarily to keep meats a fresh, reddish color. In the stomach, nitrites are converted to nitrosamines, which are carcinogenic and may raise your cancer risk. Interestingly, eating a lot of fruits and vegetables may serve as an antidote and reduce the conversion of nitrites to nitrosamines. A large-scale study has shown people who ate the most processed meats were more than 50 percent more likely to develop colon cancer than those who ate the least. To put this in perspective, though, the American Cancer Society says these dietary risks are still smaller than the risks caused by obesity and lack of exercise. If nitrites worry you, and they should, you can find processed meats made without them if you look hard enough.

While I'm on the subject of meat, cooking at very high temperatures may produce carcinogenic chemicals. It doesn't matter if the meat (or fish or poultry) is fried, broiled, or grilled. If the temperature is high enough, the heat will produce dangerous chemicals called heterocyclic amines in the meat. As a result, you should avoid the blackened parts. (Grilled vegetables and fruits do not produce the same harmful chemicals.)

When you're cooking on the barbecue, use an even heat and a lower temperature. Don't allow the flame to touch the meat. You should also consider marinating the meat or cooking smaller portions of meat, and you may want to precook meats in the oven or microwave and finish them on the grill.

Fat dripping onto coals may also produce smoke laden with carcinogens called polycyclic aromatic hydrocarbons, which lands back on the meat. So when you're grilling, try to use lean cuts of meat. Also, don't poke or press down on sausages or burgers, which can cause fat to rain down on the coals and flames to flare up toward the meat.

Artificial Sweeteners

Artificial sweeteners have produced great angst ever since the FDA banned cyclamate in 1969. Research at the time linked the sweetener to an increased risk of bladder cancer. Cyclamate remains banned, although follow-up studies failed to show a cancer link. Other sugar substitutes on the market, such as saccharin and aspartame, have also been subjected to a great deal of scientific scrutiny.

The National Cancer Institute studied about half a million people, comparing people who drank aspartame-containing beverages like diet soda with those who did not. Aspartame is sold under the brand names NutraSweet, Equal, and Canderel. The study, published in 2006, concluded that drinking more aspartame-containing beverages did not pose any additional risk of lymphomas, leukemias, or brain cancers with increased levels of consumption. It was the largest study of diet and cancer to date. The EU also concluded in 2006 that aspartame does not raise the risk of cancer.

Aspartame, which came on the market twenty-five years ago, is found not only in drinks but in thousands of other products, including chewing gum, such dairy products as yogurt, and even many medicines. (Oddly, a recent study suggests the more diet soft drinks someone drinks, the more likely that person is to gain weight, defeating the purpose of the drink in the first place.)

Studies in lab rats in the early 1970s linking saccharin (sold as Sweet'N Low) with bladder cancer prompted Congress to add a warning label: "Use of this product may be hazardous to your health. This product contains saccharin, which has been determined to cause cancer in laboratory animals." The same risk does not appear to be true in people. Population studies have not shown any compelling evidence that saccharin is linked to bladder cancer. Congress removed the warning label in 2000, the same year the U.S. National Toxicology Program removed saccharin from its list of possible carcinogens.

There are three other FDA-approved sugar substitutes: acesulfame potassium (also known as Ace-K, Sweet One, and Sunett); sucralose (sold as Splenda); and neotame, which is popular in Australia and New Zealand but new to the U.S. market. Studies have shown no evidence these artificial sweeteners pose any health risks.

In case you were wondering, artificial sweeteners are not absorbed by the body as well as sugar, which means they supply fewer calories or no calories at all. They are also significantly sweeter than sugar, so you don't have to add as much. (The makers of powdered artificial sweeteners bulk them up with dextrose or maltodextrin, a starchy powder, so they measure like sugar.) Despite the clean bill of health for artificial sweeteners, don't go overboard. As with anything we consume, moderation should be the rule.

Cell Phones

When Johnny Cochran died of a brain tumor, I admit one of my first thoughts about the famed defense attorney was the hours every day he spent on his cell phone. I have plenty of company when it comes to a gut feeling that long-term cell phone use must pose some sort of health risk. After all, holding an electronic device to your ear for long periods of time does not, on the surface, seem to be a particularly healthy way to live. But are these fears rational? Is there any science to back them up?

A large number of studies have examined whether cell phone use raises cancer risks. The intense focus is not surprising. After all, cell phones do produce a small amount of radiation. With more than a billion cell phone users worldwide, even a small risk affects a lot of people.

Almost all of the studies to date have failed to show any link between cell phones and cancer. A few Swedish studies suggested extensive, long-term use of cell phones increased the risk of a type of brain tumor called an acoustic neuroma, a benign tumor of the nerve linking the ear to the brain, in the ear usually used for phone calls. But subsequent studies have found no relation between cell phone use and the incidence of these acoustic neuromas.

The American Cancer Society says the consensus among well-designed population studies is that "there is no consistent association between cell phone use and brain cancer." The World Health Organization (WHO) concludes that cell phones are "unlikely to induce or promote cancers." Researchers with the European Institute of Cancer Research concluded there is no substantial risk of an acoustic neuroma in the first decade of cell phone use, but did not rule out an increased risk over a longer period.

The British government has urged a "precautionary approach" and advised British subjects to keep call times short. The British guidelines also recommend that children under sixteen limit cell phone use to essential calls only, which seems to be the height of wishful thinking.

Keep in mind, cell phones are a relatively new technology, so the health effects of a lifetime of use are not known.

The greatest immediate danger from cell phone use is distraction behind the wheel, even for drivers using a hands-free device. The science here is clear. If you talk on a cell phone while you're driving, you greatly increase your chance of having an accident.

Food and Plastics

Maybe you've gotten the e-mail warning you of the dangers of heating food in plastic containers or using plastic wrap. They have gained quite a bit of currency on the Internet. But will microwaving plastics really cause carcinogenic dioxins to leach into your food? The answer to this question is a definitive no. That's because there is no dioxin in these plastics. Another e-mail that has made the rounds warns of dioxin leaching into water in plastic bottles that have been frozen. This, too, is an urban legend.

Lucky for us. Dioxins have been dubbed the most toxic compounds made by humankind and have been linked to liver damage and cancer. Most of us do have some dioxins in our body, but it's from eating animals that have ingested the pollutant. We also have traces of a number of other compounds. For the most part, these appear to be harmless in the minute amounts present in our bodies.

Let's take the microscope to a pair of chemical compounds that have been the legitimate focus of scientific concern: phthalates and bisphenol-A (BPA).

Phthalates (THA lates) are used to make plastic and vinyl more flexible and their scents and colors last longer. They are used in cosmetics, medical equipment, raincoats, and toys. Phthalates are animal carcinogens, and scientists say they have the potential to disrupt hormones in humans. Because children may be at greater risk from exposure to phthalates, the United States and Canada prohibit these compounds from infant bottle nipples, teethers, and toys intended for mouthing. The European Parliament in 2005 voted to permanently ban three phthalate compounds in all children's toys and three more in toys that can be put in a child's mouth.

BPA is an ingredient in the hard, clear plastic used for bicycle helmets, sunglasses, water bottles, "sippy" cups, microwave cookware, and other products. Research suggests some BPA leaches from food or drink containers with extensive use. The American Plastics Council counters that the amount is so miniscule, BPA does not pose "a risk to human health." The FDA, which assesses the safety of food and beverage containers, agrees, saying on the FDA Web site they are "well within the margin of safety based on information available to the agency." Also, a published review of fifty studies conducted from 2002 to 2006 concluded that "the weight of evidence does not support the hypothesis that low oral doses of BPA adversely affect human reproductive and developmental health."

Not all the news is good for BPA. Like phthalates, BPA is considered an endocrine disrupter, mimicking the female hormone estrogen and potentially increasing the risk of breast or prostate cancer. One recent study found BPA sped the growth of breast and ovarian cancers in a test tube. Another study, in rats, linked early exposure to BPA with cancer of the prostate. Of course, what happens in the lab and to rats does not necessarily predict what will happen in humans. Even so, the U.S. Environmental Protection Agency (EPA) has started the Endocrine Disruptors Research Initiative.

San Francisco is not waiting for the results. Beginning in December 2006, San Francisco banned anyone from selling or distributing toys or baby bottles containing BPA to children under three. The city also banned pacifiers, toys, and children's raincoats containing some phthalates.

To be safe, look for sippy cups made from polyethylene or polypropylene. Also, don't use take-out containers or reused margarine tubs in the microwave. Only use plastic or plastic wrap that is labeled "microwave safe" in the microwave. (If you buy food with instructions telling you to put the container in the microwave, then the plastic packaging has been tested and is deemed microwave safe.) Safer still, you can use inert containers, such as heat-resistant glass or ceramic.

Even if you slip up and use plastic that is not microwave safe, you will not ingest a dangerous amount of plastic with one mistake. Just don't make a habit of it.

Teflon

A DuPont scientist discovered this revolutionary compound almost seventy years ago, but recently concerns have been raised about the safety of Teflon and other nonstick materials used in everything from grease-resistant packaging to waterproof garments to stain-resistant carpet. An estimated 95 percent of Americans have detectable levels of Teflon-related chemicals in their blood.

Perfluorooctanoic acid (PFOA), a substance used to make Teflon, causes cancer in laboratory animals and is classified as a likely human carcinogen by the EPA. Here's a sobering fact: The FDA found that the grease-resistant coating on the inside of microwave popcorn bags breaks down during microwaving, leaving traces of PFOA in the popcorn oil.

On Teflon-coated cookware, DuPont says PFOA fumes are released only when pans become extremely hot, more than 660 degrees Fahrenheit (340 degrees Celsius). More than a dozen lawsuits filed against DuPont claim Teflon releases PFOA at much lower temperatures, even during normal cooking.

Federal officials say there is no reason to stop using Teflon and other nonstick coatings because their levels in our blood are very small, and there is no proven link between these substances and cancer in humans. If you are cooking with nonstick pots and pans, you should play it safe and cook at a lower temperature. Also, never put them over heat when empty. One last piece of advice: don't microwave greasy food in a cardboard container, which is likely to be lined with a nonstick coating.

Cancer Myths

Let's dispense with a couple more myths that you might run across on the Internet. A great deal of research has been devoted to the effects of fluoride in water, toothpaste, and dental treatments. The conclusion: fluoride does not raise cancer risk. Food additives also have not been shown to increase your chance of getting cancer. Antiperspirants and deodorants, too, do not raise your cancer risk, according to the National Cancer Institute and the FDA.

EAT YOUR VEGETABLES

T. Colin Campbell, a professor emeritus of nutritional biochemistry at Cornell University, spent twenty years studying how different diets in different regions of rural China affected cancer rates. Because nine in ten Chinese live out their lives near their birthplace, rural China is an ideal "living laboratory," to borrow Campbell's phrase. Cancer rates varied from region to region more than one hundredfold. His conclusion: as many as 80 percent to 90 percent of all cancers could be prevented until very old age by adopting a plant-based diet.

The American Cancer Society, too, has increasingly been looking at improving diet and increasing exercise as a very real way to prevent cancer. A third of all cancer deaths—about

188,000—are attributable to too little exercise and not enough healthy food, according to the American Cancer Society. More than a third of Americans get no leisure time physical activity, and more than three-quarters do not eat the recommended five fruits and vegetables a day. What is especially worrisome, the organization says, is the increase in the number of overweight children, who frequently become obese adults.

A diet rich in fruits and vegetables lowers the risk of cancers of the mouth, esophagus, lung, stomach, colon, and rectum. Ideally, your diet should be rich in dark, leafy vegetables and brightly colored fruits and vegetables. Whenever possible, avoid heavily processed foods, choosing instead whole or minimally processed food. Avoid fat. Pick foods low in salt. Finally, evidence is growing that eating food from animals increases our cancer risk. As someone who enjoys a good steak now and then, this is disheartening. Most Americans—and I include myself in this group—eat too much meat. Cut down on how much meat you eat, and you will likely cut your cancer risk. I have already started, and I now limit myself to a steak or burger once a month.

Exercise is the other half of the cancer-prevention equation. According to the American Cancer Society, thirty minutes of exercise five days a week reduces the risk for breast and colon cancer, and more exercise may be better. For example, physical activity either at work or during leisure time is associated with a 50-percent reduction in your chance of getting colon cancer. Obesity, on the other hand, increases the levels of the hormones estrogen and insulin circulating in the body, which can stimulate cancer growth.

EARLY DETECTION

A number of tests exist to screen for cancer before you are experiencing any symptoms. Making sure you get these tests is vital to reducing your chances of dying from cancer. There is a universal truth in medicine: catch it early, and you are more likely to beat it. Unfortunately, many Americans fail to follow recommended cancer screenings for colorectal, cervical, and breast cancers. Detecting these cancers early means catching them at their most treatable phase. For example, diagnosing breast cancer at its localized stage means a five-year survival rate of 97.9 percent. In the case of colorectal and cervical cancer, screening can prevent the occurrence of cancerous cells altogether. Precancerous polyps, in the case of colorectal cancer, and precancerous lesions, in the case of cervical cancer, can be detected and treated.

For people who are not experiencing any symptoms, the American Cancer Society recommends yearly mammograms starting at age forty. Clinical breast exams should also be administered about every three years for women in their twenties and thirties and annually for women forty and older. Women with a family history, genetic tendency, or previous breast cancer should talk with their doctors about beginning mammograms earlier. Women who notice any change during a breast self-exam should contact their doctor immediately.

A woman should begin undergoing annual Pap smears for cervical cancer about three years after she begins having vaginal intercourse, but no later than age twenty-one. The alternative is a liquid-based test every two years. Parents of girls as young as nine may also want to speak with their doctors about a cervical cancer vaccine, which was FDA approved in the summer of 2006. After age thirty, women with three normal tests in a row can get screened every two or three years. Women seventy and older can stop cervical cancer screening altogether if they have had three normal Pap tests in a row in the previous decade.

Beginning at age fifty, men and women should be tested for colon and rectal cancer, according to the American Cancer Society. Among the options: an annual fecal occult blood test (FOBT) or fecal immunochemical test (FIT); a flexible sigmoidoscopy or double-contrast barium enema every five years; and a colonoscopy every ten years. People who are at a high risk because of a family history or some other factor should talk to their doctor about a different testing schedule. Tragically, at least 50 percent of the people who should be getting tested are not. By not getting tested, they are needlessly raising their risks of dying of cancer. Catching colon cancer early, when it is most treatable, gives you a 90 percent chance of survival five years beyond diagnosis. If you are one of those people too embarrassed to talk to your doctor about getting tested or simply do not want to undergo the test itself, you should think of the alternative.

Beginning at fifty, men should also begin screening for prostate cancer. That means an annual digital rectal examination and a prostate-specific antigen (PSA) test. Men at high risk—African Americans and those with a strong family history—should begin testing at age forty-five.

At menopause, the American Cancer Society recommends all women be warned about the risks of endometrial cancer and told to contact their doctors immediately if they experience any unexpected spotting or bleeding.

Finally, don't underestimate the annual physical. During it, your doctor should feel for enlarged or abnormal lymph nodes, thyroid gland, and (depending on your gender) testes and ovaries. Dentists now routinely check for signs of cancers of the mouth.

Sun Protection

One other way to reduce your chance of dying of cancer is to protect yourself in the sun. Almost all skin cancers are the result of unprotected and excessive exposure to the sun's ultraviolet (UV) radiation, yet less than two-thirds of all adults say they are likely to protect themselves from the sun, according to the National Cancer Institute.

The American Cancer Society estimates that UV exposure is associated with more than 1 million cases of basal or squamous skin cancers and more than 62,000 cases of malignant melanoma in 2006. If you became sunburned as a child, you have a greater risk of melanoma or other skin cancers. Light skin color, the presence of moles or freckles, and a personal or family history of melanoma also increase your chances of this skin cancer.

This won't come as a surprise, but sunblock, wide-brim hats, avoiding direct sun in the middle of the day, and avoiding tanning beds and sunlamps are all ways to significantly lower your risk of skin cancer. If you are a parent reading this, you should make sure your kids are protected when they go out into the sun. No matter what your age, you need to reapply sunblock often.

DELAYED DETECTION

Seven in ten women now undergo mammograms to check for breast cancer, a figure that has more than doubled since 1987. Still, there are far too many people who simply forgo a visit to the doctor, even when they have developed significant problems. Sometimes, it takes the illness of someone famous to remind us to get to the doctor's office. After the tragic news of the death of Peter Jennings and then Dana Reeve, the number of calls to quit smoking hotlines went up by 50 percent. It seems that all smokers and former smokers were suddenly very worried. Micki McCabe is a case in point. We met up with her in New York City. She watched the coverage about Peter Jennings and, as a former smoker, decided to get her own cough checked out. Initially, she received antibiotics for that nagging cough, because doctors thought it was pneumonia. When that didn't work, she had X-rays and then a computed tomography (CT) scan. This last test detected tumors—lung cancer. McCabe was glad she paid attention and was motivated to act after watching the tragic stories of Jennings and Reeve. Her cancer was detected early enough that an operation was able to remove all of it.

Of course, most of us never want to get to the point where we need surgery in the first place. Eating more fruits and vegetables, avoiding cigarettes and other tobacco products, and limiting alcohol consumption to one or two drinks a day help lower the chances of lung cancer—not to mention a host of other cancers.

Still, some cancers defy even the most prudent individual. There are no proven strategies for preventing cancers that arise in the bone marrow, such as multiple myeloma and leukemia.

Despite all the hype, the scientific studies on supplemental vitamins and antioxidants as cancer preventives have shown disappointing results. If you have any concern about minor deficiencies of dietary micronutrients, though, taking a multivitamin with minerals each day is cheap insurance.

All of the precautions in the world may not protect us from the assaults of time on our bodies. A common analogy among gerontologists is that once we exit our reproductive years, we become biologically irrelevant. Toxins build up; cells break down. It's not that we are designed to age. Some species die without aging. It's simply that our bodies start breaking down as the flotsam and jetsam of accumulating cellular damage start taking their toll on the basic systems in our bodies.

Many scientists believe our cells get old and die to prevent us from getting cancer. That's because DNA mutations in the cells accumulate over time as some slip by the natural processes that correct mistakes in copying our genetic blueprint from one cell to another. It should come as no surprise that most cancers occur later in life. (A seventy-year-old is about one hundred times more likely to be diagnosed with a malignancy as a nineteen-year-old.) At some point, changes in DNA result in a cell with its foot on the gas, dividing out of control—in short, a cancer cell. And here is one of the great ironies of the field of antiaging. Many who have taken on the quest to find the cure to aging look to find a way to create an immortal cell. We are already all too familiar with one such cell, a cancer cell. The same cell that could wreak so much havoc may also hold the key to our own immortality.

If you talk to any researcher studying aging about immortal cells, you will likely hear the word telomere. Turns out, a lot of research on aging has focused on telomeres, which are at the ends of our chromosomes. They shorten each time our DNA divides. When the telomeres get short enough, they stop dividing, and cellular senescence begins. Interestingly, researchers have found the telomeres of centenarians are generally long. The telomeres of an immortal cell may never shorten; they may never age. On the flip side, researchers have also found that chronically stressed individuals—for example, parents of chronically ill children—have shorter telomeres, on average, than do others their age.

It is true that cancer is one of the biggest killers in the world and one of the greatest obstacles in our quest to chase life together. Remember, though, you don't have to resign yourself to simply getting cancer and suffering if you are diagnosed. Starting today, there are things you can do to fend off the onslaught of toxic forces trying to unravel your DNA and shorten your telomeres. They are simple things and are incredibly effective, if you take the time to practice them.

Richard Nixon, who himself died of a stroke at the age of eighty-one, tried to leave his mark on history as the president who ended cancer. Unfortunately, more than thirty-five years later, cancer is still with us. But many significant battles have been won in the war against "the beast."

Paging Dr. Gupta

- ✓ Regular screening and early detection are the best ways to never hear the word cancer.
- ✓ Don't ignore symptoms. Pick up the phone and call your doctor.
- ✓ Eat five to seven servings of fruits and vegetables every day.
- ✓ Separate fact from myth. Get the details on Teflon, beef, cell phones, artificial sweeteners, and plastics.
- ✓ Know the nine controllable cancer risk factors—you *can* lower your risks.
- ✓ Exercise more and cut down on fat, salt, and animal products.
- ✓ Help protect your telomeres by lowering your stress level.

CHAPTER 7

A Growing Problem

What if I said just by looking at you, I could tell whether you had an elevated risk of heart disease, stroke, and diabetes? I wouldn't need to take a blood test or know your cholesterol level. I wouldn't need to know any facts about your lifestyle or diet. I wouldn't need to take a family history. In fact, I wouldn't need to say a word to you. All I would need to do is give you a quick glance. What I would be doing is checking your waist size. How big you are around the middle now is a harbinger of health problems down the road.

To be more precise in my diagnosis, of course, I would use a tape measure. Think about it, though. In this age of high-tech medicine, of CT scans and MRI machines, a tape measure may be the best diagnostic tool we have to predict your risk of heart disease, stroke, and diabetes. That's because your waist size shows how much abdominal fat your body is carrying. Abdominal fat, it turns out, is a killer.

How large a waist is dangerous? According to the National

Obesity Forum, a waistline of thirty-five inches or more for women and forty inches or more for men should sound the alarm. That's because people who are large around the middle—with a so-called apple-shaped body—tend to have more fat not just on the outside, but more importantly surrounding and choking the internal organs. People who have fat on their thighs or buttocks—pear-shaped bodies—have more of their fat stored just under the skin. Not surprisingly, having more visceral fat—fat stored around the internal organs—is far more dangerous. Put simply, a big stomach is much worse for your health than big hips. Men are more likely than women to be apple shaped, although visceral fat is also a risk for postmenopausal women.

As a doctor, I am always looking for ways to actually show people what all that extra abdominal fat is really doing to the body. That is why I was so fascinated by an exhibit traveling the globe with specially treated human cadavers. It is called Body Worlds: The Anatomical Exhibition of Real Human Bodies, featuring more than two hundred human specimens ranging from entire bodies to individual organs. A German named Dr. Gunther von Hagens took cadavers donated by individuals from all over the world. The skin has been removed so you can see the bones, tendons, muscles, nerves, blood vessels, and healthy and diseased organs. All of the natural fluids in the body have been replaced with a flexible plastic, a process invented by von Hagens and dubbed plastination. The process is designed to stop decay after death, offering some truly unique and somewhat gruesome views of the human body.

One body in the exhibit has been sliced down the middle, from head to foot. Others are posed playing chess, running, jumping, fencing, kicking a soccer ball, and swinging a baseball bat. One body is even posed atop a preserved horse. Seeing these skinless "plastinates" posed as if performing ordinary activities is both shocking and fascinating.

More than 16 million people have seen Body Worlds in Europe and the United States. In an effort to find out how I might live longer, I decided I should see the specially preserved cadavers firsthand. I caught up with the Body Worlds exhibit at the Franklin Institute Science Museum in Philadelphia. The goal of Body Worlds is to promote healthy lifestyles, and it is easy to see why it might work.

Because you can peer into the wonderful complexity of the human body, you can see the differences in the bodies on display. There is a cadaver of a person who weighed 580 pounds near someone who weighed 140 pounds. The difference is truly striking. The first thing that hits you is all the extra weight that person carried around. It's not surprising, for example, that this body had an artificial knee. The wear and tear of all that extra weight takes its toll on the joints, which have not evolved to carry around excess pounds.

Then you look at the organs. You can actually see the fat on the liver of the overweight cadaver. A fatty liver won't work as well as a healthy one, and that will affect the body's ability to flush out toxins and deal with the waste products of the body's metabolism. Even the heart is not immune. It is immense: three or four times normal size. Fat has gotten into the heart tissue itself, weakening it. Fatty buildup in arteries also makes people more prone to blockages, causing heart attacks.

Looking at the bodies in Body Worlds left me with a lasting impression and little doubt in my mind that globs of fat around the midsection are far more dangerous than simply causing your pants to be snug. That is the bad news.

This book, however, is about chasing life, so I have good news as well. Fat around the waist appears to be the easiest to lose, far easier than fat on the hips or buttocks. In fact, a study at Duke University Medical Center found a brisk half-hour walk six times a week could stop the waistline from expanding any further. If you can find time for even more exercise, you could actually start to reduce the visceral fat. It goes without saying that doing no exercise resulted in increased abdominal fat and about 4 pounds a year of weight gain.

As you have already learned, chasing life means lowering your risk of heart disease, stroke, and diabetes. These are the biggest killers in most developed countries, but if you follow some fairly simple steps, we can cut your risk dramatically and greatly extend your life. Unlike many books out there, I won't make you the false promise of a magic formula, and I will demand your full participation. But trust me—the payoff will be well worth it. The first step is to start today—I mean right now.

True, you may be decades away from any chance of heart disease or stroke, but remember, the way you live now will most certainly have an impact on your health in the future. Diabetes is a good example. Type 2 diabetes used to be synonymous with adult onset, but now, because of poor choices at a very young age, we are seeing this type of diabetes in grade school children. More about that later.

HEART HEALTHY

We know more about heart disease today than ever before. Heart disease is the number-one killer in the United States, accounting for 2.4 million deaths, according to the most recent figures available. That's 1 in every 2.7 deaths, or almost 2,500 Americans a day. That's more than the next four leading causes of death combined (cancer, chronic lower respiratory diseases, accidents, and diabetes). Of course, this is nothing new. Since 1900, heart disease has caused more deaths than any other cause every year except 1918, when the worldwide flu pandemic swept through the United States. Unfortunately, heart disease shows no signs of going away anytime soon.

Some 71 million Americans now suffer from one or more types of cardiovascular disease, more than two-thirds of them under the age of sixty-five, according to the 2006 statistics from the American Heart Association.

Heart troubles tend to get worse with age. For example, high blood pressure hits a little more than 20 percent of Americans in their forties, 60 percent of Americans in their sixties, and 80 percent of Americans in their eighties. African Americans are more likely to be affected. Researchers have found that the stiffness of blood vessels increases as we age, when flexible fibers are replaced with less flexible collagen and calcium. This process thickens the interior wall of the blood vessels and raises blood pressure. Researchers are now trying to figure out ways to stop this vascular aging. Exercise helps. Arterial stiffness is inversely related to physical fitness.

From remarkable medications to invasive procedures, doctors have become good at treating heart disease. But as we chase life, it is important to get control of the risk factors to your heart before you are ever diagnosed with full-blown heart disease. This is especially true if you have a family history of heart troubles. Yes, you want to start off with a visit to your doctor's office, but you want to go armed with knowledge. Here are some of the basics: Make sure you know your family history well. Pay attention to any unusual pain in your chest, especially if it's crushing or radiating into your jaw or arm, so you can tell your doctor about it. If you have ever had your blood pressure checked or had an electrocardiogram (EKG) in the past, make sure you take that information with you, as well as previous cholesterol readings. This can save you a lot of time in the doctor's office and make sure you are off to a good start. Too often, I have heard stories of a patient whose first symptom of heart disease is a heart attack. And, given that one-third of all heart attacks are fatal, it is often both a surprising and disastrous outcome. Obviously, you want to catch potential problems like high cholesterol, cardiac arrhythmias, and atherosclerosis—a buildup of plaque in the arteries—before they reach the critical stage. Sometimes it's not as easy as it sounds. Former President Bill Clinton experienced eight years of executive health care while in the White House. Still, that wasn't enough to stave off life-threatening heart disease just four years later, when he went under the knife to have heart bypass surgery. "I really think it probably saved my life," Bill Clinton told me, speaking not about the bypass operation he had but about the test—an angiogram—that first showed that the arteries feeding blood to his heart were dangerously blocked. "If people have a family history there, and high cholesterol and high blood pressure," Clinton said, "they ought to consider the angiogram."

Good advice? Yes and no. An angiogram is the gold standard of heart tests, and in Clinton's case, it picked up a problem that all his previous stress tests and EKGs had missed. But an angiogram is not something to be taken lightly. It involves injecting a dye directly into the blood vessels of your heart through a catheter that has been threaded into your chest from an artery in your groin. By taking X-ray images of the dye, doctors can get a pretty clear picture of where blood is flowing freely and where there are constrictions.

But angiograms are not risk-free. In about one case out of one thousand, according to Dr. Richard Stein, associate chairman of medicine at Beth Israel Medical Center in New York City, there are complications—including, in rare cases, strokes. For patients who have never had any symptoms (such as the chest pains and shortness of breath that Clinton experienced) and whose stress tests are normal, the risks outweigh the benefits, says Stein.

That's why there has been so much attention given lately to a noninvasive test called electron beam computed tomography (EBCT). It uses a burst of X-rays to show how much calcium has been deposited in the coronary arteries—a good measure of how much plaque has accumulated there. In a study published in the *Journal of the American College of Cardiology*, more than half of 1,119 patients who passed their stress tests had high calcium scores in subsequent EBCTs, suggesting significant hardening of the arteries.

Getting an EBCT is not the end of the story. If you get a high calcium count, you will still need an angiogram so your doctor can tell precisely where your arteries are blocked. But EBCTs are spotting a lot of hidden heart disease. Although some insurance companies are reluctant to pay for this new test, its use is growing rapidly, and it may eventually become part of the standard heart workup. This is something you may want to talk to your doctor about if you have a strong family history of heart disease or have other reasons for concern.

There has also been a lot of interest in a new sort of blood test called C-reactive protein (CRP). President Bush has his checked regularly, and it is extraordinarily low, which means to him (and his doctors) that he is at very low risk of having a heart attack. At medical cocktail parties nowadays, it seems cardiologists are talking about CRP the way they used to talk about high-density lipoprotein (HDL) and low-density lipoprotein (LDL), and for good reason. Two recent reports from the *New England Journal of Medicine* suggest that CRP may be just as important a risk factor for coronary artery disease and heart attacks as LDL—and maybe more so. CRP is a protein secreted by the liver in response to inflammation, and over the past several years, it has become apparent to experts that inflammation is a big part of heart disease. CRP seems to play a role in damaging artery walls, making them more prone to the buildup of fatty plaques that can rupture and block the vessels that feed the heart. Sure enough, studies have shown that high CRP levels, signaling active inflammation, are significantly associated with heart problems. So what can you do about it? Well, doctors know statins can reduce inflammation. So cardiologists from Brigham and Women's Hospital in Boston put 3,745 patients who had experienced heart attacks or severe chest pain on statins and later measured their levels of both LDL and CRP. It turned out that patients who ended up with low CRP levels were less likely to have heart attacks or die than were those whose CRP levels stayed high—whether or not their LDL levels went down. This was in many ways a landmark study, showing that CRP reduction is at least as important as cholesterol reduction. The second study, performed at the Cleveland Clinic Heart Center, also tracked cardiac patients, but instead of looking at heart attacks, the researchers measured actual plaque buildup. The patients whose CRP level dropped the most while taking statins saw their plaques get smaller—again, independent of what happened to their LDL level. There is no question that CRP will continue to become increasingly important, and it now makes sense for anyone who's at risk for heart disease to be evaluated. It's a simple blood test that any lab can do, and while it might not be covered by all insurance companies, it costs $15 at most.

Still, for us life chasers, I want to start with the basics so we may never need these medications, tests, or operations. It comes down to working out harder, sleeping more soundly, and being very particular about what and how much you eat.

Exercise

Exercising is the first simple step toward lowering your risk of heart disease. If you become leaner and fitter, your risk of heart disease and stroke goes down. It's that simple. Not exercising raises your risk of coronary artery disease as much as high blood pressure, high cholesterol, or smoking, according to a study published in the *Journal of the American Medical Association*. You also know that focusing on losing that abdominal fat makes a world of difference. So in addition to such aerobic activities as running, stair climbing, or perhaps walking on a treadmill, you want to do some targeted, core exercises to work off that abdominal fat. As you gradually add even small amounts of weight training to your program, you will start to see the abdominal fat melt away. And here is an added benefit: it will also likely help you get critically important, quality sleep at night.

Sleep

Chronic lack of sleep has been linked with heart disease, among other health problems. A number of studies have linked sleep with appetite and weight control. One study, involving more than one thousand people between the ages of forty-five and seventy-five, found the body mass index (BMI) of participants actually increased as their sleep time decreased. I know it seems counterintuitive, but it turns out the less you sleep, the more your overall metabolism changes, conserving energy and fat. So lack of sleep makes your fat that much harder to lose and thus contributes to heart disease. In another study, researchers restricted young, healthy adults to four hours of sleep a night for six days and found some remarkable, measurable hormonal changes that could lead to overeating. The study subjects actually developed decreased levels of leptin, an appetite suppressant. And to make matters even worse, they had increased levels of ghrelin, a hormone that stimulates appetite.

Smoking

If you smoke, you should stop. If you don't smoke, please don't start. It's amazing that with all the information out there about the horrible health consequences of breathing in cigarette smoke, an estimated 1.4 million Americans start smoking each year (half of them under eighteen). You must know the association between smoking and cancer, but those nasty nicotine-delivery devices also result in an estimated doubling or tripling of your risk of dying from coronary artery disease, according to the American Heart Association. I am not going to preach about cigarettes, although I recently learned not enough doctors counsel their patients to quit. Let me simply say that everything else in this book is null and void if you continue to smoke or ever start.

Nutrition

There are certain foods that appear to help protect against heart disease. I call them "power foods," and you should try to incorporate as many as you can every day into your diet. A large-scale study found a diet high in fruits and vegetables and low-fat dairy products; with moderate amounts of fish, poultry, and nuts; and low in red meats, sweets, and sugary drinks lowered blood pressure by as much as seventeen points in people with high blood pressure. And that was within just two weeks. In case you ever thought simple changes to your diet wouldn't amount to much, think again. Cholesterol also dropped within that same time period.

Despite this straightforward antidote, the statistics collected by the American Heart Association are extremely worrisome. For example, four in five men and nearly three in four women do not get the recommended five servings of fruits and vegetables a day. A third of our calories come from fat, and our diets are low in whole grains. Our daily fat consumption is about 75 grams, the equivalent of three McDonald's Quarter Pounders with cheese. In a very real way, we are by and large what we eat—fat.

Eating a fatty diet is so easy in the United States. Fast food restaurants, vending machines, and gas station marts offer up food that is high in fat. Even hospitals are offering fatty fare. A study commissioned by the Center for Science in the Public Interest found cafeterias at eighteen of the nation's top hospitals were serving foods prepared with partially hydrogenated vegetable oil, the biggest source of artery-clogging trans fat in the American diet.

Heart Disease Power Foods

- Fruits, especially strawberries, blueberries, and bananas
- Vegetables, including tomatoes, spinach, eggplant, and okra
- Low-fat dairy
- Legumes such as lentils, chickpeas, and lima beans
- Fish, especially such oily fish as tuna, mackerel, and herring
- Poultry
- Nuts, including almonds and walnuts
- Whole grains

Here are some heart-healthy foods: such oily fish as tuna, mackerel, and herring, which contain omega-3 fatty acids, can significantly lower the risk of dying of heart disease, according to the American College of Cardiology.

Eating foods containing soluble fiber, such as oat bran and legumes, has been shown to lower total cholesterol and LDL (bad) cholesterol. Blueberries may have a similar effect. Lycopene, found in tomatoes and tomato products, such as ketchup and tomato juice, may also lower cholesterol and reduce the risk of heart attack, although results from a number of studies are not consistent. Okra and eggplant have also been shown to lower cholesterol, as long as they are not fried.

Adding strawberries to your diet could lower your systolic blood pressure.

One study found eating cereal fibers later in life lowered the risk of cardiovascular disease. This is one area in which Americans really fall short. The recommended daily intake is 25 grams, but we are averaging about 15.

A heart risk you don't often hear about comes from the amino acid homocysteine. Elevated levels of homocysteine in the blood increase the risk for such cardiovascular diseases as coronary artery disease, stroke, and blood clots. That's true even for people with normal cholesterol levels. In fact, high homocysteine levels account for an estimated 10 to 20 percent of cases of coronary artery disease and pose as big a threat as high blood pressure and hypertension. Fortunately, there appears to be a simple dietary fix.

Adding folic acid, or folate, to your diet decreases the homocysteine levels in the blood, which should in turn lower the risk of heart disease and stroke. How do you increase your folic acid intake? The simplest sources of folic acid are fortified breakfast cereals and folic acid supplements. Green, leafy vegetables, such as spinach, are rich in folic acid, as are citrus juices and legumes, such as lentils, chickpeas, and lima beans. In addition, heavy drinkers, cancer patients, and pregnant women all need extra folic acid in their diets.

The minerals we get in our food also affect our heart health. The National Health and Nutrition Examination Surveys, which involved nearly ten thousand men and women whose eating habits were charted for two decades, revealed that those who had the lowest potassium levels in their diet had a 28 percent greater risk of stroke than those who consumed more potassium-rich foods. The Honolulu Heart Program, which studied seven thousand men, found those with the highest magnesium intake had a 45 percent lower risk of heart disease than did those who consumed the least.

Good sources of potassium include bananas, baked potatoes, orange juice, raisins, prunes, and spinach. Sources of magnesium include bran cereal, oat bran, shredded wheat, brown rice, almonds, hazelnuts, almonds, spinach, okra, lima beans, and bananas.

In a year-long study conducted by the University of Toronto, something called the portfolio diet showed cholesterol-lowering properties that rivaled the blockbuster cholesterol drugs known as statins. The diet allowed for no meat, eggs, poultry, fish, or dairy. Foods were picked based on their ability to lower cholesterol a little. Together, they lowered cholesterol a lot. What was it? Participants in the study ate a mostly vegetarian diet also rich in soy foods, almonds, and fruit. They also ate whole grains and beans, and they used healthy oils and margarine made from plants.

Another study found omega-3 fatty acids, which I talked about in chapter 5, reduced the chance of dying of heart disease more than statins.

STATINS, SUPPLEMENTS, AND OTHER DRUGS

Dr. Steve Nissen, a cardiologist at the Cleveland Clinic, told me we are almost to the point in the United States where we should put the class of cholesterol-lowering medications called statins in the drinking water. "The medications are that good," he added. I am pretty sure he was exaggerating somewhat, but not that much. Nissen is not alone. Many doctors consider statins a true wonder drug.

Truth is, most people do not rely on dietary changes, but instead take drugs to lower their cholesterol. An estimated 20 million Americans now take cholesterol-lowering statins. One of these drugs, atorvastatin (Lipitor), is the best-selling drug in the world. Despite their popularity and their effectiveness at lowering cholesterol, you should try lowering your cholesterol through dietary changes before you take one of these drugs—unless you're cholesterol is dangerously high.

Not everyone is enthusiastic about the widespread use of statins to prevent heart disease. Dr. John Abramson, who teaches primary care at Harvard Medical School, argues in his book *Overdo$ed America* that statins are widely overprescribed, thanks to a recommendation made in 2001 by an influential panel of experts. The guidelines they published suggested increasing the number of Americans who qualify as having cholesterol levels high enough to warrant statins from 13 million to 36 million, and doctors have largely followed these recommendations. But Abramson argues that the gradual buildup of plaque in the arteries caused by cholesterol is not the main cause of heart attacks. Rather, he says, it is when a small area of plaque breaks open, triggering first a blood clot and then a heart attack. The cause of these "fractures" is not known.

Abramson recommends prescribing statins for people who

already have coronary artery disease, but not for patients with only moderately elevated cholesterol levels, and he says a number of large trials back him up. Despite his criticisms, there appears to be no letup in the number of prescriptions written for statins.

Before you start taking statins, be aware that the drugs have rare but significant side effects. The drugs can cause muscle weakness and raise liver enzymes.

More than 20 million Americans take aspirin to help prevent heart attacks and strokes. Aspirin's benefits as an anticlotting drug have been known for decades, but the latest research suggests that the situation is not as clear-cut as once believed.

For starters, recent studies suggest from 1 million to more than 8 million of these aspirin users do not get the drug's anticlotting benefits. They are aspirin-resistant and will not reduce their chances of heart attack or stroke by taking the drug. The findings do not affect people who take aspirin for inflammation or pain.

Most doctors who advise their patients to take aspirin do not test for aspirin resistance, although new tests make it easier than ever to do so. The alternative to aspirin to lower the risk of heart attack or stroke is a popular antistroke drug called clopidogrel bisulphate (Plavix), which is far more expensive.

In addition to resistance, there appear to be some differences in the way men and women respond to aspirin. A ten-year study of healthy women found taking low-dose aspirin did not prevent first heart attacks in women younger than sixty-five.

Aspirin does help men under sixty-five. In fact, one study of healthy men showed taking an aspirin pill every other day reduced their risk of heart attack by 44 percent.

Because aspirin can cause bleeding, doctors recommend only men and women at risk for heart disease take aspirin for this purpose. Risks include a family history of heart disease, high blood pressure, or diabetes. Anyone over sixty-five is also considered at risk for heart disease.

Even with its potential to cause bleeding, aspirin is less likely to cause ulcers than Plavix, a recent study published in the *New England Journal of Medicine* found. Patients on Plavix suffered from ulcers more than twelve times as often as did people who took aspirin plus a heartburn pill. This countered the conventional wisdom that Plavix was safer for the stomach than aspirin.

An estimated 23 million Americans take vitamin E, many of them no doubt in an effort to prevent heart disease. As I noted in chapter 3, studies have not backed up the efficacy of this behavior.

DIABETES

Being overweight doesn't only raise your risk of heart disease, it also puts you squarely in the crosshairs of diabetes. Diabetes is linked to a host of serious physical complications. They include heart disease, stroke, high blood pressure, blindness, kidney disease, gum disease, damage to the nervous system, and tissue death that can necessitate amputation. Diabetes has so many complications, it has been likened to the aging process itself. It is a disease that can shorten your life span and prematurely age your body. If you are serious about chasing life, you must try to prevent diabetes from ever taking hold in the first place and diligently control your blood sugar if it does.

An estimated 70 percent of your risk of diabetes in the United States comes from being overweight. Given the growing girth in this country, it follows that the number of diabetics in this country is skyrocketing.

The American Diabetes Association estimates 20.8 million Americans are now diabetic, with nine in ten of the cases being type 2 diabetes. With type 2 diabetes, the body does not produce enough insulin or does not properly use insulin, a hormone needed to convert sugars, starches, and other food into energy. Obesity complicates the situation by increasing both blood sugar levels and insulin resistance.

More than 6 million Americans don't even know they have diabetes, according to the American Diabetes Association. Signs you are diabetic include increased thirst, hunger, fatigue, and urination (especially at night); also, blurred vision and sores that do not heal. If you are forty-five or older and overweight, you should get tested for diabetes. Your doctor will check your fasting blood glucose level. Make sure to ask about this if you are concerned.

You have a higher risk of diabetes if you are a minority, have a family history of the disease, have high blood pressure, have low HDL ("good") cholesterol, or do not exercise much. Women who had gestational diabetes or gave birth to a baby weighing more than 9 pounds are also at higher risk.

In general, diabetes becomes more common as we get older, but the obesity epidemic in this country is putting more and younger adults at risk. Some 41 million Americans have a condition called prediabetes, in which blood sugar levels are higher than normal, but not high enough to warrant a diagnosis of diabetes.

As I wrote, the numbers appear to be even more troubling for this country's minorities. The number of African Americans aged forty to seventy-four with diabetes more than doubled in the last decade, according to statistics reported in a federal health survey. The prevalence among blacks is now approaching twice that of whites. Hispanics, too, are disproportionately diabetic. The rate of diabetes among Hispanics is almost twice that of whites of similar age, according to the CDC.

The number of diabetics in the United States is expected to more than double in the next twenty years. By some estimates, one in four Americans will be diabetic in the year 2025.

Weight

Lifestyle plays a critical role in developing type 2 diabetes. Just like with heart disease, eating a healthy diet and exercising are crucial for avoiding diabetes. What's more, waist circumference also appears to be a good predictor of type 2 diabetes. As with heart disease, waist circumference appears to be a better predictor than body mass index, or BMI. BMI is simply the ratio of your weight in kilograms to the square of your height in meters.

Even moderate weight loss combined with exercise can

lower blood sugar and improve insulin sensitivity, helping to prevent the development of full-blown diabetes. According to one estimate, if you are overweight and lose 5 percent to 7 percent of your body weight through diet and exercise, you can cut your risk of getting diabetes by more than half. For example, if you weigh 250 pounds and lose just 12.5 pounds, your blood sugar level will go down and your insulin action will be improved.

Nutrition

In general, if you are at risk of getting diabetes, here are some simple tips. First off, you should really pay attention to portion control. Then, limit your fat intake to about 25 percent of your total calories. Also, eat more fruits and vegetables.

Here is something I found fascinating. A very low fat, vegetarian diet appears to be very beneficial for diabetics. More than a third of those who had been previously treated with insulin were able to stop the medication after switching to this diet. At the same time, blood sugar and cholesterol levels dropped. Researchers who tracked a group of more than twenty-five thousand Seventh-Day Adventists for twenty-one years found diabetes was lower among vegetarians than the others.

Even if you are not a vegetarian, increasing the number of fruits and vegetables and lowering the amount of saturated fat in your diet will help cut your chances of developing diabetes. As with heart disease, eating whole grains, nuts, soy proteins, and such cereal fibers as barley and oats appears to reduce the risk of diabetes. If you are confused about the best diabetic diet, you are not alone. You may have heard that foods ending in *–ose* (like *lactose*) or *–ol* (like *sorbitol*) are an absolute no-no. Well, that is not necessarily the case. And to take it one step further, you don't have to restrict yourself to sugar-free foods only. Yes, you can eat sugar, even as a diabetic. As with most things, though, moderation is the key, along with sensible food choices.

First off, a couple of definitions. The *–oses* that you hear about are naturally occurring sugars; fructose, for example, is the sugar found in fruits. The *–ols* are the sugars found in alcohols. The reason diabetics pay so much attention to this is sugar and carbohydrates can be difficult to process. During digestion, a healthy person's body converts carbohydrates from food into various sugar molecules. These sugars are further converted, mainly into glucose, the primary fuel used by the body. With the aid of insulin (a hormone produced by the pancreas), glucose enters cells to provide the body with energy.

But in people with type 2 diabetes, either the pancreas doesn't make enough insulin, or the muscles and other tissue have become resistant to insulin, or both. As a result, sugar accumulates in the bloodstream, causing all sorts of problems, from fatigue to numbness to even kidney problems or blindness.

As a result, it was believed for most of medical history that a diabetic should avoid eating all sugars. But over the last decade, smart doctors and dieticians have challenged the traditional diabetic diet. What really seems to matter, it turns out, is how the diet overall incorporates carbohydrates. If you are someone concerned about diabetes, it is more important to pay attention to the type of carbohydrates you eat and the frequency with which you consume them than it is to avoid all sugars.

You can reduce your risk of diabetes by eating "better" carbohydrates. Carbs are the body's main source of energy. They are sugar molecules and break down into glucose. Carbohydrates that break down more quickly cause a spike in blood sugar and can raise your risk for diabetes (and heart disease). Carbs that break down more slowly cause the smallest fluctuations in blood sugar.

Spikes in blood sugar are bad because they require your pancreas to produce a surge of insulin. Over time, spikes in blood sugar will cause our bodies to become less sensitive to insulin. The end result can be diabetes.

So what are "good" carbs? Carbohydrates are classified using a scale called a glycemic index. This scale measures how far and how fast our blood sugar rises after eating a certain food that contains carbohydrates. The scale ranges from 0, the healthiest carb, to 100, the least healthy.

Foods containing refined sugars and corn syrup have a very high glycemic index. For example, the average donut has a glycemic index of 76. Unfortunately, most Westerners eat far too many foods loaded with high glycemic carbs. Processed foods also tend to have a very high glycemic index. White bread has a glycemic index of 71 or more. French fries have a glycemic index of 75. By contrast, fruit like apples, oranges, and grapes have a low glycemic index, as do many beans. Brown rice, oat bran cereal, whole wheat bread and spaghetti tend to be in the middle.

If you want to check the glycemic index of a specific food, go to glycemicindex.com, a site run by scientists and dietitians at the University of Sydney. If you want to switch to a low glycemic index diet, the folks at the University of Sydney recommend eating breakfast cereals made from oats, barley and bran; eating bread made from sour dough, whole grains or stone-ground flour; reducing the amount of potatoes in your diet; and switching from white rice to basmati or brown rice.

Futurist Ray Kurzweil claims he has been able to cure his type 2 diabetes by eliminating all high glycemic carbs from his diet. He says cutting them out of his diet was easier than simply reducing the amount of high glycemic carbs in the food he ate.

"If you don't stop eating starches and sugars as a significant part of your diet, you're going to continue to have these cravings. If you really adopt a sharp reduction in those, the cravings go away," Kurzweil told me in an interview.

I'm not recommending that you eliminate carbohydrates from your diet, just that you lower the glycemic index of the carbs you do eat.

The information given in *The Joslin Guide to Diabetes: A Program for Managing Your Treatment* and *16 Myths of a Diabetic Diet* is based on these simple facts. According to experts at the well-known Joslin Diabetes Center, you can have a piece of cake on your birthday and go out to dinner. You just need to know how to count carbohydrates and sometimes limit certain foods. By the way, this advice is also useful if you simply want to lose weight.

Also, in case you are wondering, artificial sweeteners are not all the same. Be careful when you are selecting the best artificial sweeteners. "Sugarless," "sugar-free," and "no-sugar-added" can all have very different meanings that are important for diabetics. There are nutritive or caloric sweeteners, such as sugar alcohols, that add calories and affect blood glucose levels. Then there are nonnutritive or noncaloric sweeteners, such as aspartame, sucralose, saccharine, and acesulfame potassium, which, after extensive testing, are regarded as safe for the general public, including diabetics.

Controlling Diabetes

- Maintain a healthy weight.
- Eat a healthy diet containing plenty of fruits and vegetables.
- Exercise regularly.
- Limit your fat intake and control your portion sizes.
- Count your carbohydrates.

Today, with all we have learned about nutrition, diets, and carbohydrates, the diabetic diet has undergone an overhaul. It is probably better not to avoid all sugars altogether, but to think about eating a certain number of carbohydrates throughout the day—just not all at once. So, for example, you can have a few peanut M&M's as long as you cut back on sugar elsewhere in your diet.

And so what about those *–ols*? On first blush, sugar alcohols may sound like a good thing for diabetics. After all, they are lower in calories than regular sugar, and the body absorbs them more slowly, resulting in a slower rise in blood sugar. Keep in mind, however, that foods containing sugar alcohols usually contain many other ingredients that contribute calories, and that sugar alcohols can have a laxative effect. So make sure to read all the ingredients when buying these foods. As you can see, there really is no such thing as an absolute diabetic diet, and diabetics don't have to be relegated to eating boring and tasteless foods. Just follow some simple rules.

Future

There is no question that carrying around too much weight pushes us backward in our quest for longer life. If you are forty years old and even moderately overweight, say good-bye to more than three years of life. If you have crossed over into obesity, you will lose nearly a decade. Think about that—losing nearly ten years of life for what is a very fixable problem. First off, remember what happens too often in our food-rich, exercise-poor society. When you combine a lot of calories with a sedentary lifestyle, the pancreas needs to kick into high gear to produce enough insulin to dispose of the excess blood sugar. Over time, this excess blood glucose results in visceral fat. Eventually, this leads to an altered metabolic state in which you are producing very high levels of insulin, but the body is less sensitive to it. The result can be diabetes, high blood pressure, kidney disease, and heart disease.

Because food was not a sure thing in more primitive times, our bodies developed the ability to hang onto every calorie we consumed. In fact, there is an actual gene in our body, a sort of insulin receptor gene that is always telling our body to hang onto fat and store it in our midsection. This insulin receptor gene was great news when we were hunting and gathering our food. It protected us against starvation during a bad hunting season. Now that getting enough food is not a problem for most people living in the developed world, the insulin receptor gene has become a big problem. While our society has evolved, certain aspects of our bodies have not. But what if we could turn off this gene? What if we were able to help the body compensate for the high calories and couch potato lifestyle? What if we could help clear away the excess blood glucose before it was turned into fat—before we started down the road to obesity, diabetes, and heart disease? One day, we will likely have that ability. Scientists around the world are looking at how exactly this gene might be altered so that obesity and associated heart disease, stroke, and diabetes become things of the past. I get asked about the future a lot when I talk about health and fitness. It is true that in the coming years, science may be able to give us the potential benefits of eating a calorie-restricted diet without the pain. I promise you that when that day comes, I will make sure you know all about it. Luckily for you, we don't have to wait for that day. Now that you have a better understanding of how heart problems, stroke, and diabetes develop, you can start making some simple changes in your everyday choices to help you chase life.

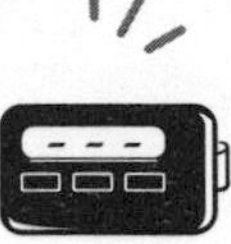

Paging Dr. Gupta

- ✓ Get rid of that apple-shaped midsection.
- ✓ Visit your doctor armed with knowledge. Know your family history and the tests you may need to detect heart disease and diabetes.
- ✓ If your cholesterol level is out of control, strongly consider switching to a healthier diet (that includes blueberries, tomatoes, okra, and eggplant) and a statin medication.
- ✓ Get plenty of sleep. It will help you lose weight.
- ✓ Eat smarter. Increase the amount of "power foods" in your diet.
- ✓ A little weight training could provide big results—and great abs.
- ✓ Know your CRP levels—it's more important than you may think.

CHAPTER 8

Sunny-Side Up

Leonard Abraham was born in Tarrytown and has lived all of his ninety-five years in the picturesque village north of New York City. His sons have long since grown and moved out. His wife has died, leaving Abraham alone in the house he has lived in for more than four decades. Still, the retired engineer says he is not lonely. He keeps in touch with his large extended family. He reads. He gardens. He has traveled the world and says he would still like to take a cruise in South America, the one continent he has not visited.

"I still have all my marbles, so I don't consider myself too old. If my body would move as fast as my mind, it would be very good," he told me.

Abraham credits his long life to genetics. His mother died at 102, his father at 85. However, within minutes of meeting him, I could easily see that Abraham shares a trait with many of those who live into very old age: an upbeat disposition. Those who make it into their nineties and beyond seem to be able to cope with hardships better than most, to adapt to the curveballs life throws, to maintain an interest in learning new things, and to exude a positive attitude. They are usually upbeat and open to new experiences even though many have endured seemingly crushing personal tragedies and physical hardships.

Abraham makes all his own meals and eats well. He cooks fish several times a week and eats plenty of vegetables. In this day and age, when master suites are usually built on the first floor, Abraham's bedroom is on the second, and the ninety-five-year-old gets up and down the stairs without much difficulty. In fact, Abraham has been active his whole life. He played community volleyball until he was seventy-five and mowed his lawn into his nineties. His life has not been without vices, though. He smoked cigarettes until he was forty-five or fifty and gave up cigars only two years before we met. He drank alcohol but has given up all but the occasional beer on the advice of his urologist.

On an average day, Abraham says he gets up and reads the papers. He waters the garden if it needs it. He does his own laundry once a week. He visits his neighbors. He no longer restores vintage cars, but he still likes to drive, and he has chosen a car you might associate with a much younger man—a PT Cruiser. The silver car sat spotless in his driveway when he invited me to come visit. Abraham also remains passionate about his other hobby, photography. He proudly showed me photographs he has taken of family and places he has visited. I spent a day with Leonard Abraham, and in that short time, I could already feel my disposition improving and my outlook becoming a little brighter.

Attitude seems to make a difference. Baseball Hall of Fame pitcher Satchel Page, who played major-league baseball into his fifties, once asked a great question: "How old would you be if you didn't know how old you were?" As we chase life, we should ask ourselves Page's question carefully—and answer honestly.

Remember Jeanne Calment, the Frenchwoman who lived to be 122? At her 120th birthday party, a journalist reportedly told her, "Well, I guess I'll see you next year."

Without hesitation, she is said to have replied, "I don't see why not. You look to be in pretty good health to me."

But can optimism—a good attitude about life and aging—help you live longer? That's where I am headed in this chapter.

OPTIMISM IS OPTIMAL

First, let's consider what neuroscientists have been learning about the brain recently. For years, the brain was thought to be immutable. We were born with a certain number of brain cells, which were wired during our formative years and gradually flickered out as we approached senescence.

Now, such brain imaging techniques as function magnetic resonance imaging (fMRI) are teaching neuroscientists that the brain is always changing, building new pathways, newer connections. In fact, our brains form a million connections every second. Neuroscientists call the ever-changing nature of our brains neuroplasticity. The ramifications of this new understanding of the brain are huge. It means the way we live our lives—our social interactions, emotions, and environment—can produce profound and long-lasting changes in our brains' structure. The brain, in turn, sends signals to the body, which regulates, for example, hormone production. As we'll see, our mental life—how we perceive the world—can affect our body in significant and not always beneficial ways. A bleak outlook can have very real physical consequences.

You've probably heard stories about a longtime husband or wife who died of "a broken heart"—a spouse whose death followed his or her partner's by days or weeks. An epidemiological study funded by the National Institute on Aging found that the death of one spouse increased the risk of death of the other spouse by 21 percent for men and 17 percent for women in the next two years. That's compared with others in that age group who didn't lose a partner.

The same study shows how even a serious ailment in one spouse can result in catastrophic health consequences for the other. Interestingly, it wasn't the most deadly diseases that had the most dramatic effect on the health of the caregiving spouse. Certain cancers, for example, didn't increase the risk of death for the partner at all. Husbands of women hospitalized for pancreatic or lung cancers had a lower risk of death, even though those cancers are particularly deadly. The hospitalizations that produced the highest risk of death of the caregiving spouse were dementia and psychiatric disorders. They produced a higher mortality risk than a partner's death. The reasons for this weren't addressed in the study. Perhaps these mental ailments were so hard on the spouse because of the social consequences of the illnesses. The husband and wife were no longer able to interact as a couple.

If you don't think your outlook on life has a real, physical effect on your brain, consider this study: Scientists looked at how people who experienced a trauma early in life responded to positive and negative images and compared that to a control group. What they found was that those who had experienced an early trauma, such as the loss of a parent, had a muted response to the positive images and a heightened response to the negative ones. Researchers also found structural differences in the hippocampi of these two groups. As you may remember from chapter 5, the hippocampus is a horseshoe-shaped structure in the center of the brain that is involved with memory formation and learning.

So, if your life can change your brain, can a positive outlook help you live longer? Can optimism help you live a longer life? The answer appears to be a resounding yes. A study published in the *Journal of Personality and Social Psychology* in 2002 found that longevity is increased dramatically by positive self-perceptions of aging. Researchers from Yale and Miami universities checked the National Death Index against residents of a small Ohio town who had been surveyed twenty-three years earlier about their perceptions of aging. When these 660 Ohioans were surveyed originally, in 1975, they were fifty or older, "cognitively intact," and residents of the same unnamed town of 15,000.

Researchers asked these Ohioans to answer "yes" or "no" to the following statements: "Things keep getting worse as I get older"; "I have as much pep as I did last year"; "I am as happy now as when I was younger." They were also asked to fill in the blank in the statement "As I get older, things are (better, worse, the same) as [sic] I thought they would be." The answers were assigned values, and the scores were tabulated.

When the researchers looked at what happened to these folks more than a quarter of a century later, the results were astonishing. Those with a more positive self-perception of aging lived 7.5 years longer, on average. This advantage remained after the researchers had controlled for age, gender, socioeconomic status, loneliness, and functional health. Those with a better outlook on aging demonstrated better survival rates regardless of their age—even if their health was worse than others in the group.

The results were not a fluke, either. Dutch researchers followed more than five hundred men aged sixty-four to eighty-four for fifteen years. At the outset and twice more during the decade and a half of the study, researchers asked each of the men whether they fully agreed, partly agreed, or did not agree with the following statements: "I still expect much from life"; "I do not look forward to what lies ahead for me in the years to come"; "My days seems to be passing by slowly"; and "I am still full of plans." How they answered these questions allowed the researchers to determine the "dispositional optimism" of the study participants. The men who were optimists when the study began, in 1985, were 55 percent less likely to die of heart disease or stroke by the time the study ended, in 2000. You might think a family history of heart problems or people in poor health would produce pessimists and result in a higher rate of heart disease or stroke. You might also speculate that pessimists are more likely to be cigarette smokers, which also significantly raises the risk of death from cardiovascular disease. But the Dutch researchers calculated their results after taking into account these risk factors. Optimists somehow did a far better job of avoiding the West's number-one killer.

The authors had no scientific explanation for the startling results, published in the *Archives of Internal Medicine* in 2006. They were left to speculate why optimists did so much better. Perhaps optimists are better at coping with adversity or take better care of themselves when they get sick. Others have suggested optimists are more likely to live healthy lives and enjoy greater social support.

A study of medical outpatients in Minnesota found similarly dramatic results. Thirty-five years after they were asked to take an optimism-pessimism personality test, the pessimists were "significantly associated" with poorer self-reported physical and mental functioning and had an overall lower survival rate. Even if you are a pessimist by nature, you can act like an optimist. That alone will make you more likely to take action, become informed, and seek out solutions.

Of course, I don't want to confuse a very important point. Your attitude on life is different from depression, which is a clinical condition that could require medication. If you are depressed, wishful thinking won't help. You should see a doctor.

OUTLOOK AND LONGEVITY

But if optimism and a positive outlook help, how does it work? That is something that has puzzled researchers, but British researchers have found a few clues. They started with two possibilities. First, as I already mentioned, positive well-being could be associated with favorable health habits and lifestyles. In other words, people who felt good about their lives took care of their bodies. On the flip side, people who were not happy about their lives would engage in unhealthy behaviors. Cigarette smoking, the researchers noted, is associated with psychological distress, and those who are anxious or depressed are less likely to exercise.

The second possibility is that someone's outlook on life could affect biological systems such as immune responses, through the central nervous system. The researchers measured heart rate and blood pressure throughout the day. They also measured the stress hormone cortisol (in saliva) every two hours and asked people to rate their happiness on a scale of one to five every twenty minutes. Here is what they found: the happier the individual said he or she was, the lower the heart rate and the lower the cortisol level.

The U.S. Department of Health and Human Services conducts a survey that looks at the flip side of the coin: asking how often Americans experience feelings of sadness, worthlessness, and hopelessness. The federal agency found 3.2 percent of all Americans said they were sad all or most of the time. Women were sad almost twice as often as men. Women were also much more likely than men to experience a feeling of worthlessness all or most of the time (2.3 percent to 1.5 percent).

Survey Says?

Just how happy are we in the United States? A 2006 survey by the Pew Research Center found 34 percent of Americans are very happy. Another 50 percent say they are "pretty happy," while 15 percent say they are "not too happy." For those of you who did the math, the last 1 percent said they "didn't know" if they were happy.

According to the survey, marriage tends to make us happier (equally for men and women). So does worshipping regularly. Healthy people tend to be happier. So do college graduates. Republicans are happier than Democrats. Both are happier than independents. Whites and Hispanics are happier than blacks. People who live in the Sunbelt are happier than those living in the rest of the country. And those of us who are "always" rushed report being less happy than others who only are "sometimes" or "almost never" rushed.

Surprisingly, we tend to get happier as we get older. Young men (age eighteen to twenty-nine) are the least happy group, according to the Pew survey, while men sixty-five and older are the happiest. The Pew survey found parents are no happier than people with no children, once you control for marital status. Also, once we've met our basic needs of food and shelter, money does not buy much happiness. But the Pew survey found those who made the most money ($150,000 or more) were more likely to report being "very happy." I am convinced it may have less to do with money and more to do with attaining a sense of accomplishment in their field.

Sadness was also highest in the Northeast and among divorced or separated individuals (even higher than among the widowed). Midwesterners and people who were married were least likely to be sad. Interestingly, Northeasterners were the saddest, collectively, but they were the least likely to feel worthless all or most of the time. That distinction fell to Southerners.

All of this raises a chicken and egg question. Are people happy because they graduated from college and embarked on a successful career, or is it the other way around? Do people get through college and embark on a successful career because they are happy? Is it possible that for many of us, happiness breeds educational and financial success and not the other way around? That's something Sonja Lyubomirsky, of the University of California, Berkeley, and fellow researchers decided to investigate. Previous research looking into happiness and success tended to assume that success led to happiness, and not the other way around.

To question this basic assumption, Lyubomirsky, along with Laura King of the University of Missouri and Ed Diener with the Gallup Organization and the University of Illinois at Urbana-Champaign, examined the connections between life successes and well-being in more than 275,000 people. They did this by examining the findings from three different kinds of studies—225 studies in all: longitudinal studies, which follow the same group of people over a period of time; cross-sectional studies, comparing different groups of people;

and experimental studies, changing variables under controlled conditions to see what happens to measured results.

The researchers concluded that happy individuals are more likely to seek out and undertake new goals. This, in turn, reinforces positive emotions. Happy individuals, they concluded, are also more likely to have fulfilling marriages, high incomes, superior work performance, community involvement, and robust health.

"Study after study shows that happiness precedes important outcomes and indicators of thriving, including fulfilling and productive work, satisfying relationships and superior mental and physical health and longevity," Lyubomirsky and her coauthors wrote in an article published in *Psychological Bulletin*.

Consider this: Academy Award winners live 3.9 years longer on average than do those who were nominated but did not win. Donald Redelmeier, a professor of medicine at the University of Toronto, did the math. He found Oscar winners in lead and supporting roles live an average of 79.7 years. The "losers" live an average of 75.8 years.

Happiness in and of itself is not a magic pill that ensures good health. After all, the king of the Himalayan nation of Bhutan makes public policy decisions based on how they will effect what they call the Gross National Happiness, but Bhutan's life expectancy—sixty-one years for men and sixty-four years for women—is far less than that of the United States (seventy-five years for men and eighty years for women) and other industrialized nations.

Nor is optimism alone a surefire route to long life. Africans are the most optimistic people on the planet, according to Gallup International, but this bright outlook has unfortunately not spared the continent's residents from miseries including starvation, HIV, and a sadly short life span.

STRESSED OUT?

So what exactly is the connection between happiness and a long life? Increasingly, researchers believe the link between optimism and good health is related to stress. If you are one who sees the glass as half full or sees setbacks as challenges to overcome, you probably feel less stress than someone who sees the glass as half empty and sees setbacks as things that are out of his or her control. At the Mind Body Medical Institute in Chestnut Hill, Massachusetts, the mission is to help people improve their health by reducing the destructive stress in their lives. The institute has special programs for people with cancer, chronic pain, heart disease, and other ailments, such as asthma and allergies.

"Between 60 and 90 percent of visits to the doctor are related to stress," says Dr. Herbert Benson, the president of the Mind Body Medical Institute, a professor of medicine at Harvard, and the author of the 1975 best-seller *The Relaxation Response*. Benson has spent more than forty years looking beyond traditional medicine to the power of the mind as a powerful tool.

"Stress cannot be avoided" Benson told me when I visited

him on a beautiful June day underneath an impossibly blue sky. In fact, "Stress is getting worse and worse. We give people an approach to specifically counteract stress." Benson's approach does not come in a bottle or require a prescription. He harnesses the power of the mind with what he calls the relaxation response, the physiological opposite of the stress response.

First, let's define stress here as an overwhelming physical or mental challenge—or the expectation of one. Fear and uncertainty cause stress. Highly competitive environments cause stress. So does change, even when it is change for the better. Stress is in the eye of the beholder. What causes it for one person may not cause it in another. One person may find driving on the highway stressful while another calmly flies a helicopter in a war zone. Our attitude about life can influence how much stress we feel in a given situation. Faced with the same set of facts, an optimist may see an opportunity, while a pessimist sees only problems. By the same token, optimism or confidence will help us perceive a problem as something that can be overcome. Pessimism or a lack of confidence can make the same problem seem insurmountable.

Stress can affect every aspect of your life, but it is not always bad. Stress is a natural part of life, and it can help motivate us. For example, I thrive on a certain amount of stress, and challenges seem to fill my life, although I now know these constant stressors may be shortening my life span. Performing brain surgery and serving as the chief medical correspondent for a major international television network each carry a level of stress I crave. Others might find operating on the brain or appearing on camera incredibly stressful—regardless of training or ability (40 percent of Americans fear public speaking, more than fear heights or flying).

What exactly is going on in our bodies when we experience stress? First of all, our bodies are designed to respond to stress in much the same way an animal's does. When we perceive stress, we prepare our bodies to fight or flee. We are stronger, quicker, and more alert than normal. We've all heard the story about the woman lifting the car to free her trapped child or the severely injured man walking miles to find help. The body is really capable of remarkable things when survival is on the line.

So how does this fight-or-flight response work? It's really incredibly logical. If you need speed, strength, and alertness immediately, you need energy. To get that, your body sends signals to fat and muscle cells. You also need to deliver this energy as quickly as possible. To do that, a surge of epinephrine (adrenaline) and norepinephrine causes your breathing, heart rate, and blood pressure to increase, helping to move these nutrients and oxygen around your body as quickly as possible. Other stress-related changes during the fight-or-flight response are the blunting of pain and the improvement of memory. These are all clever ways your body reacts to help you survive a life-or-death situation.

There are also systems in your body that are not crucial for immediate survival, so the body slows them down or puts them on hold. For example, digestion and the immune response are inhibited, and sex drive decreases.

So it also seems logical that being stressed all the time is not good for our bodies. The fight-or-flight response is designed to help us deal with a relatively quick confrontation or crisis. It is not meant to be activated for the long term. For one thing, if we are stressed all the time, our bodies are constantly speeding short-term energy to our muscles. That means we won't store any surplus energy. As a result, we are likely to get tired more easily. Because it changes our metabolism, stress also raises our risk of getting diabetes. If your heart rate and blood pressure are constantly elevated, you are putting strain on the cardiovascular system and raising your risk of high blood pressure, cardiac irregularities, and heart attack. If you suppress your immune system for too long, you are more likely to contract an infectious disease. Ever wonder why you get the sniffles at the end of a particularly hard week at work? Other stress-related ailments include ulcers, allergies, asthma, migraine headaches, and obesity. As we learned in chapter 5, stress also raises the risk for Alzheimer's disease. Stress can also contribute to infertility and make premenstrual syndrome (PMS) and other existing medical conditions worse.

STRESS-BUSTERS

For reasons great and small, then, it is important to reduce the stress in our lives. No doubt, this is easier said than done.

There are healthy ways to deal with stress. They may even be enjoyable. Some people find exercise an excellent way to relieve stress. Others use meditation or prayer to bring calm into their lives. Even sitting at your desk and taking deep breaths or closing your eyes tightly with your mouth closed are said to be stress relievers. Others recommend yoga, massage, soothing music, or a warm bath. Talking to a friend or a counselor or writing about your stress are said to help. So is sex.

To avoid stress, try an attitude adjustment. Even on a busy day, take a moment to slow down and relax. Think of stressful situations as challenges, not as threats. Consider the worst-case scenario and the chances of that happening. Determine what you can control and whether you have done everything possible to change the outcome.

Benson's Mind Body Medical Institute teaches patients how to induce the relaxation response, an activity he says has its roots in the earliest civilizations. As a result, you can harness the power of thought, he says, to lower your blood pressure, heart rate, metabolism, and rate of breathing to bring on feelings of clarity and well-being.

Benson says we can trigger the relaxation response by following our breathing in and out and breaking the train of everyday thought. He says we can do this through repetition: repeating a word, a sound, a prayer, or a movement. We can do this through meditation, prayer, yoga, tai chi, or jogging, he says, adding quickly that there is hard science to back up everything he recommends. In fact, the latest neuroscience shows brain scans of people who meditate actually show less aging than those who don't.

Benson, who looks like a kindly minister, gave me a demonstration of his relaxation technique. First, I chose a word I was comfortable with: gentle. Each time I exhaled, I repeated the word. I have to admit, as tightly wound as I normally am, I was a bit skeptical that this would work. Still, I really let my mind go exactly where the good doctor was taking it. After about five minutes of this, Benson observed my facial muscles were noticeably more relaxed. Even though it was just a few minutes, when I slowly opened my eyes, it felt as if I had been resting for an hour. Shutting off the mind like this, Benson says, helps the body revert to its natural healing state.

"We can effectively treat many forms of hypertension, anxiety, mild and moderate depression, insomnia, PMS, many aspects of infertility. They can all be effectively treated by a mind body component to our modern medicine when needed," Benson told me.

And Benson says it shouldn't come as a surprise that many "aha" moments come when we are far from our stressful, competitive environment—in the shower, taking a walk, at the gym. Many of our best ideas come when our minds are free to wander.

In addition to contributing to physical ills during the day, stress also gets in the way of sleep. Some 50 to 70 million Americans have trouble getting to sleep or staying asleep at night. Many of us wake up in the middle of the night, worried about things left undone. Stress keeps us awake, and the fatigue the following day only adds to our stress.

MIND AND BODY

Have you ever started feeling better the moment you called the doctor's office to set up an appointment? If so, you're not alone. The symptoms remain, but you are less worried about them, so you feel better. Having a doctor really listen to you may add to your sense that you are improving. Studies have even shown that if you undergo simple diagnostic procedures, you are more likely to have a better outcome than patients who do not have these tests performed.

If you have any doubt about the powerful effect of the mind to summon our own healing powers, consider the placebo. A placebo is usually a sugar or otherwise medically inert pill masquerading as a real drug. Most hospitals ban the use of placebos, and most doctors frown on using them, because it involves lying to patients. Yet many physicians believe inert medicine can work.

In clinical trials, patients are divided into two groups. One group gets the drug under consideration. The other group gets a sugar pill, a placebo. Neither the study participants nor the doctors administering the drug know which is which. This makes the study "double blind." Nothing in the pill or the way the pill is administered could tip off the participant. A review of fifty-two clinical trials for depression found the placebo did better than the antidepressant more than half the time. The antidepressant only did better than the placebo in 48 percent of the cases, although the antidepressant did work better with severely depressed people.

Placebos have effects that are not only in the mind. Some studies show placebos produce physiological changes. In one study, doctors painted warts with a bright but inert dye and told patients the warts would be gone when the color wore off. They were. In another, researchers found they could open the airways of asthmatics simply by telling them they were inhaling a bronchodilator.

Placebo Surgery?

Diseases are one thing, but how about placebo surgery? What if patients underwent sham surgeries for arthritic knees? How would they fare, compared with those who received the real thing? Dr. Nelda Wray of the Houston VA and Baylor College of Medicine decided to find out, with the help of Dr. Bruce Moseley, a clinical associate professor of surgery at Baylor College of Medicine and team doctor for the Houston Rockets and Houston Comets basketball teams.

Moseley operated on a total of 180 patients with osteoarthritic knees. Some of them received arthroscopic surgery, while others received placebo surgery—a small incision and nothing else. Two years later, those who received the sham procedure felt just as much pain relief—

and sometimes more—than those who had the standard scraping and rinsing of the knee joint. They also reported just as much improvement in joint function.

Six months after the procedure, doctors asked participants if they wanted to have the surgery done on the other knee. Twelve said yes. Of those twelve, six were with the placebo group. Needless to say, more than a few orthopedic surgeons were not happy with the study's conclusions and defended arthroscopic knee surgery for patients with arthritis.

The study was not a ringing endorsement for the $5,000 knee surgery, which is performed on more than two hundred thousand people a year. It does say a lot about the potential power of the placebo effect, though.

Their findings mirror the results of a University of Kansas study conducted in the 1950s, in which doctors performed real and sham surgery for angina pectoris, or chest pain. A perfect 100 percent of patients receiving the bogus operation said it helped with their symptoms, compared with 76 percent who underwent the actual surgery.

Two brain imaging studies concluded placebos work in much the same way as the real thing. Injections of bogus painkillers activated the brain's natural painkillers (endorphins), while clinically depressed patients taking a placebo experienced brain activity in the same part of the brain as those taking antidepressants.

Some skeptics have called the placebo effect a myth, claiming that no treatment at all will succeed in treating some diseases, simply because the illness has run its course. Either that, or the placebo effect is exaggerated or simply the result of chance. A patient who feels ill one day is bound to feel better the next. Benson at the Mind Body Medical Institute says there is too much evidence to discount the placebo effect.

Doctors who believe in the healing power of placebos say much of the placebo effect may come from the doctor-patient interaction itself. The placebo is not an absence of treatment, the reasoning goes, simply an absence of active medication. The act of receiving treatment and believing the treatment will be beneficial has—at least in some cases—the power to heal.

The brain is not always an ally, though. If you have ever listened closely to the drug ads on television, they usually end with a list of potential side effects, such as headaches, nausea, or fatigue, and then add, "about the same as the sugar pill." That means the test subjects in the placebo group experienced side effects from an inert pill. This is what researchers have dubbed the nocebo effect. *Nocebo* is Latin for "I will harm." It is often called the evil twin of *placebo*, Latin for "I will please." With a nocebo effect, if test subjects believe there may be side effects, they often experience them. Again, expectations shape reality.

A British study testing a chemotherapy drug against a placebo in stomach cancer patients found that a third of the placebo recipients lost their hair, and a fifth developed nausea and vomiting. An Australian study looking at anabolic steroids had placebo recipients complaining of steroid-induced acne and the irritability often referred to as "'roid rage."

This leads me back to the way our outlook can profoundly influence our health and well-being. Part of this may be because there are ten times as many nerves carrying information from the brain as there are sensory nerves giving information to the brain. The brain takes the sensory information and makes sense of it. Top-down processing would make sense of the power of placebos or nocebos. If the mind is convinced, the senses will be ignored. Signals from the brain also appear to influence our physiology in profound ways. The brain can interact with the body by controlling hormones and through the nerve pathways to control everything from heart rate to immune function.

The mind—your mind—is an incredible weapon at your disposal. Your attitude about the world can have a very real physiological effect. Stay upbeat, and your brain may tune your body to help you live longer. Maintain a sour disposition and a negative outlook on life, and your health may well be adversely affected.

I don't know how long Leonard Abraham will live, although he invited me to his next birthday party. And I doubt he ever consciously decided to improve his disposition because he wanted to live longer. Yet Abraham teaches us something profound. Despite all the advancements made in the field of longevity, it is our mind that may still hold some of the greatest weapons. We have only begun to scratch the surface of learning to harness the power of our minds over our bodies, but we do know that power can be magnificent. So are you curious about what the future might hold? Well, let's continue our chase for life into the future.

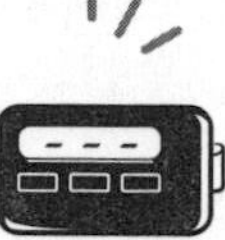

Paging Dr. Gupta

- ✓ Practice optimism. It can help you have a longer life.
- ✓ Spend a few minutes every day relaxing or meditating. A few deep breaths can do wonders.
- ✓ Allow your mind to slow down and wander several times a day.
- ✓ Avoid stress; try an attitude adjustment.
- ✓ Ask yourself how old you would be if you didn't know how old you were.
- ✓ If you are depressed, get treated. It will be good for your mind and your body.

CHAPTER 9

The Future Is Coming

Ray Kurzweil is doing everything he can to live long enough to see the future. To get there, the fifty-six-year-old subjects himself to an unbelievably rigorous diet and health regimen, popping 250 supplements a day and washing them down with green tea. The author and inventor is constantly testing himself—measuring his progress with an array of tests, from reaction time, memory, tactile sensitivity, and such biochemical markers as hormone, vitamin, and nutrient levels in his body. When he first started testing himself seventeen years ago, Kurzweil says, he tested like someone who was thirty-eight. Now, he says, tests show he has the body of a forty-year-old. By his calculations, his biological age has advanced two years, while his chronological age has marched ahead seventeen years.

That's just the beginning, according to Kurzweil, who invented the first reading machine for the blind and has been inducted into the National Inventors Hall of Fame. The futurist predicts if he lives ten to fifteen more years, he will be able to take advantage of the full flowering of the revolution in knowledge of the human body; maximum life expectancy, now around one hundred years, will start extending out decades and decades. Jeanne Calment, the Frenchwoman who made it to 122, will not be the exception. She won't even be the rule. People in developed countries will routinely exceed her mark, with the help of scientific breakthroughs that are currently on the horizon.

Kurzweil has spent much of his life ahead of the curve. As a teenager in 1965, long before advent of the personal computer, he appeared on the Steve Allen show *I've Got a Secret* for writing a computer program that composed music. The MIT graduate, now the chairman of Kurzweil Technologies in Wellesley, Massachusetts, also invented the flatbed scanner and the first commercial speech-recognition software, among other things. Kurzweil is not alone among forward-thinking researchers in his belief that science will start increasing the human life span. But with his books and speaking engagements around the country, he is perhaps the most vocal. His two most recent books tout the coming revolution: *The Singularity Is Near: When Humans Transcend Biology* and *Fantastic Voyage: Live Long Enough to Live Forever.*

Kurzweil speaks to packed auditoriums about the longevity boom that's right around the corner. Immortality, it seems, is a growing industry. Leading scientists have started companies with names like Elixir and Longevity. Investors, too, are buying into the possibility that the human life span can be radically altered with the help of research being done now and science not yet imagined.

Kurzweil envisions three bridges to radical life extension. We are in the midst of a biotechnology revolution, which is the first bridge. In ten to fifteen years, we will reach the second bridge and be able to reprogram our biology to avoid cancer, heart disease, diabetes—even aging itself. By the end of the teen years, say 2019, he says, we will cross the third bridge and begin using technology at a molecular level to extend our lives significantly. We started this voyage talking about practical immortality. Perhaps you thought it far-fetched. Kurzweil thinks it is right around the corner.

"The progress in this is exponential, not linear—that's the important point," he told me, adding that the rate of scientific progress is doubling every decade. He reminds me that "it took us fifteen years to sequence HIV. We sequenced SARS in thirty-one days."

The human immunodeficiency virus (HIV), which causes acquired immunodeficiency syndrome (AIDS), began spreading in the early 1980s. Severe acute respiratory syndrome (SARS) came along two decades later. SARS, too, is caused by a virus. The first known case occurred in China in 2002 and spread to more than two dozen countries before the outbreak was contained. The ability of researchers to decode the virus so much more quickly shows the tremendous advances science has made in genetic sequencing, Kurzweil says. "Ultimately, we'll have very powerful tools to sort of reprogram our biology away from health and rejuvenate, really, all of our organs," Kurzweil told me when I sat down with him a few months ago.

Kurzweil wears very mod glasses and has a stylish haircut.

He wasn't what I was expecting when I envisioned a radical scientist, although he did jump quickly from topic to topic, letting words hang mid sentence, which gave him a professorial demeanor. In Kurzweil's brave new world, we will be the beneficiaries of personalized medicine, in which our genome will be scanned, looking for clues to future maladies. We will be able to replace our cells with younger versions of themselves. Perhaps his most outlandish prediction for the future involves microscopic robots, called nanobots, constantly circulating in our bloodstreams, reversing all known diseases and aging processes. And then there are the scientific advances coming that we can't possibly predict, because science is moving so fast. Kurzweil himself says he expects to live at least one thousand years. If that sounds crazy, you haven't sat down and listened to him.

"I think death is a tragedy. Many of our philosophies and religions have sought to rationalize that death is really a good thing. But our basic reaction is death is sad. That's it's a tremendous loss of knowledge and personality."

Eventually, Kurzweil thinks we will be able to add more than a year of life expectancy for every chronological year that passes. That means Kurzweil thinks someday, humans will be able to live forever. Kurzweil uses the example of a house. Right now, we can repair everything that goes wrong with a house. We don't have that sort of knowledge about our bodies—yet. Someday, though, he says we will be able to repair DNA and rejuvenate cells and organs the way we can fix all the systems of a house.

Unfortunately, we are far from having the same understanding of the human body as we do the systems in a house. Even unraveling the aging processes in worms and fruit flies has proven maddeningly difficult for some of the world's brightest scientists.

Then there is the debate about what lies at the root of aging. What does it mean when we talk about stopping the aging process or even slowing it? Earlier, I talked about aging as involving two components. One is more general and involves the accumulation of problems from the cells on up. Our cells stop dividing, get old, and die. Vital components in cells and tissues wear out. Our mitochondria, the power plants in our cells, become less efficient. Free radical oxygen attacks the components of our cells and causes damage. Our DNA accumulates mutations, which can lead to such serious health problems as cancer. Proteins bind together and disrupt cellular function.

The second way to look at aging is more specific. We develop heart disease. Tumors grow in our colons. Plaques and tangles accumulate in our brains. These are the signs of aging we in the medical profession try to treat when they appear. These are lumped into a category called age-related diseases. They are the kinds of problems we'd like to put off or avoid altogether, if possible.

Clearly, if we stop or postpone the diseases prevalent among the elderly, many of us would live healthier, longer lives. We would still be aging, though. The clock would still be ticking in our cells. We would risk winding up like the mythical figure Tithonus in the story dating back almost three thousand years.

The god Zeus grants Tithonus eternal life, but not perpetual youth. As a result, Tithonus lives forever, old and incoherent, locked away in a room.

ON THE HORIZON

So the obvious goal in the quest for immortality is to reach very old age with vitality. This really strikes at the heart of what we've been exploring throughout this book. We've discussed some of the basic things we can do now to help fight aging and live longer, healthier lives. The future promises much more.

In much of science, researchers try to understand a biological process by looking at it in simpler organisms first. Investigators hoping to unlock the keys of aging have done this with the roundworm known as *C. elegans*, the fruit fly, and with genetically manipulated mice. In each of these organisms, investigators have found genes associated with longer life. These genes are able to confer greater longevity by affecting stress resistance, metabolism, insulin and blood sugar levels, cell growth and survival, free radical production, and other means. To be fair, the gains sometimes come with side effects, such as dwarfism, sterility, or increased cancer risk.

A gene called *SIR2* has generated a lot of interest among researchers. Variants of the gene exist in all living organisms, from yeasts to humans. Adding a second copy of the *SIR2* gene to a yeast cell increased its life span by 30 percent. Extra copies of the gene increased the life span of the roundworm by 50 percent. Researchers believe this gene, part of a family of genes called sirtuins, may help organisms survive adversity by regulating a survival mechanism.

SIR stands for silent information regulator. The *SIR2* gene effectively silences other genes by rendering certain areas of the genetic code inaccessible. If it is activated over the long term, *SIR2* staves off disease and prolongs life. Exactly how the gene does this is not known. Even armed with this knowledge, no one has created an immortal worm or fruit fly. Not yet, anyway.

Understanding *SIR2* could someday lead to knowledge that will allow us to live longer, disease-free lives. That's because humans and other mammals have a version of the gene, known as *SIRT1*. Studies in mice and rats suggest the protein encoded by *SIRT1* allows some of the animals' cells to survive stress and enhances cellular repair mechanisms.

Remember the calorie-restricted diets I talked about in chapter 2? It appears *SIR2* is activated by calorie restriction. The stress of a calorie-restricted diet appears to cause *SIR2* activity to go up, enhancing protective mechanisms in our bodies that may help us live longer. Restrict calories in yeast, worms, or fruit flies, and *SIR2* activity increases. These organisms also live longer. If the *SIR2* gene is removed, restricting calories in these organisms has no effect on longevity.

Resveratrol (discussed in chapter 3), the substance in red wine credited with helping the French live long lives despite a fatty diet and a relatively high prevalence of smoking, also activates *SIR2*. Giving resveratrol to yeast, worms, or fruit flies increases their life spans—even without calorie restriction. In fact, resveratrol-fed fruit flies can eat as much as they want and still enjoy the benefit of longer life.

Pharmaceutical companies are researching new ways to moderate appetite, which might well help slow the aging process. Already, the drug rimonabant is on the market in Europe under the brand name Acomplia as treatment for dangerously overweight patients. Acomplia is the first of a new class of drugs designed to block receptors responsible for giving marijuana users "the munchies." FDA approval is expected sometime in 2007. Pharmaceutical companies are also investigating ways to regulate the appetite stimulating hormone, ghrelin. Even if these drugs succeed, they are not likely to be a magic bullet for weight loss. Acomplia is taken in conjunction with a diet and exercise program. Also, it is meant as a treatment for those whose weight puts them at risk for diabetes or heart disease, rather than for those who simply want to lose a few unwanted pounds.

Researchers also are studying the oldest Americans, looking for clues to their longevity on the twenty-three pairs of protein strands that form human chromosomes. They are using the latest scanning technology to look for longevity genes, something in our master code that tells our bodies not to get old, or to at least take its sweet time getting there. Although genes account for only 30 percent of our expected life span, finding a gene that could influence how long we live—or what age we get an age-related ailment, like heart disease—would be an enormous advance in living out life to its potential maximum. Understanding the genes of the very old could help drug makers produce compounds that manipulate the processes governing the aging process itself.

Looking for Longevity

Today, one in ten thousand people make it to one hundred, most of them women. The lucky few who reach the century mark often do so in remarkably good health. For starters, many often don't look their hundred years. Somehow the sands of time have moved more slowly for them. Second, many get heart disease or some other age-related disease decades later than their peers. The obvious question is why. Do they have some genetic advantage? Are they eating something with life-giving properties?

In 1998, Dr. Nir Barzilai began the Longevity Genes Project at the Albert Einstein College of Medicine in New York. Barzilai had been working with calorie-restricted animals, but he became curious about the genetic influence on life span. Barzilai and his team study Ashkenazi Jews who are 95 and older. He picked Ashkenazi Jews, because they are relatively genetically homogenous. Plagues, wars, and anti-Semitic persecution reduced their population to an estimated few hundred thousand by the seventeenth century. This relatively small group (from a demographic point of view) then experienced a rapid population growth. This small number of "founders" makes it easier to find genetic differences among Ashkenazi Jews. The genes for ovarian and breast cancer were originally discovered in studies of Ashkenazi women.

Barzilai is now looking for genetic markers for longevity in long-lived Ashkenazi Jews who are healthy and living independently. The Israeli-born doctor says he is not after the fountain of youth. He is simply trying to find ways for each of us to make the most of what we have. He thinks science and medicine have a role to play, and points to his own family as an example of how the advance of knowledge can lengthen life. His grandfather had a heart attack when he was 68 and died. His father had a heart attack at exactly the same age. Thanks to better medical care, he lived. When we spoke to Barzilai, his father was 83. Barzilai thinks humans have the potential to remain healthy past 100, possibly to 120, if he and others can figure out how to slow the aging process.

To search for genetic clues to aging, Barzilai and his team arrange for "family reunions" of those 95 and older, their children, and their children's husbands and wives. When they get family members together, they do a short physical exam and a mental test; they take measurements of height, weight, body fat, and temperature; and then they draw a blood sample. Barzilai has collected data on close to four hundred families. Blood from these families is now stored in small vials in an oversized freezer next door to his lab at Albert Einstein, in the Bronx.

What Barzilai has found is that such age-related diseases as hypertension, diabetes, heart attack, and stroke have been delayed by about thirty years in centenarians, and he is convinced genes play an important role in this delay. In fact, he says the older you get, the bigger role genes play. By the age of 100, he says, genetics is more important than environment. He has found centenarians who were obese in middle age. He has found others who smoked for more than 90 years. Literally two packs a day for more than 90 years. He has found other unhealthy behaviors these 100-year-olds somehow overcame to achieve very long life. They have defied the odds. They have avoided death and dodged disease. If their genes somehow protect them, then they should pass on those genes to their offspring. The children of the very old should also be more likely to live a long time. As you might guess, that's true. Barzilai has found the children of centenarians are generally healthier than their spouses, with whom they usually share diet and lifestyle. The New England Centenarian Study, in a separate, ongoing study of 100-year-olds, has found that centenarians are four times more likely to have a sibling who lived past 90 than is someone with an average life span.

What's behind this? Barzilai has uncovered some clues. Longevity appears to be linked to high levels of HDL ("good") cholesterol and low levels of LDL ("bad") cholesterol. Long life is more likely among those with larger HDL and LDL molecule sizes, which he says results in lower incidences of cardiovascular disease, hypertension, and insulin resistance. LDL cholesterol attaches to the vessel walls, where it can harden and turn into plaque. Over time, plaque can cause narrowing of blood vessels, raising the risk for heart disease and stroke. HDL appears to have the opposite effect, cleaning out the blood vessels. "Good" cholesterol levels typically drop with age, but not in the centenarians. Barzilai has encountered levels three times as high as expected. High levels of HDL cholesterol also appear to be linked with mental ability in very old age.

If you are interested in raising your own levels of good cholesterol, you can try drinking a moderate amount of wine, but that will cause only a very small increase in HDL, nothing at all like the levels found in Barzilai's centenarians.

In addition to what he's learned about good cholesterol levels in the very old, Barzilai has also found three genes that are overrepresented in centenarians. About 8 to 12 percent of 65-year-olds have these genes. Some 24 to 32 percent of centenarians do. Of course, this doesn't prove the genes are the cause of the longevity, but they are certainly linked with people who have achieved an extraordinary life span. People who have one of the genes appear to live four years longer than those who don't, on average. That is a huge number. If you could reproduce that gene's protective power in a pill, it would have more of an effect than would curing heart disease, he says.

Researchers conducting the New England Centenarian Study, which is also looking at genetic links to long life, pinpointed a region on chromosome 4 they believe holds at least one longevity-enabling gene. They made this discovery after scanning the genes of 137 sets of long-lived siblings.

Because women live longer, there may be a spot on the X chromosome that gives women an edge. Women have two X chromosomes; men have only one.

Barzilai believes there may be 100 longevity genes in all. Some of them might be necessary but not sufficient to promote longevity by themselves. Barzilai is currently searching centenarians' genome at 500,000 different places. By doing this, he will see which genotypes are overrepresented. There are two ways genes can help us live longer. They can slow the aging process itself, or they can protect against age-related diseases.

New Drugs

Science is also moving forward in other areas that may have profound consequences as we chase life. Something called RNA interference (RNAi) could revolutionize the way drugs work. Scientists believe it might be used someday to treat a wide range of disease and conditions, including HIV infection, cancer, hepatitis, macular degeneration, and high cholesterol.

Most medicines work by binding to the active site of a protein. This stops a chemical pathway that produces some unwanted result. Let's take the example of antidepressants such as Prozac or Zoloft. These drugs bind to receptor sites in the brain, blocking the absorption of the mood-enhancing chemical serotonin. You may have heard of these drugs referred to as SSRIs. That stands for selective serotonin reuptake inhibitors. The drugs stop the reuptake of serotonin, keeping the levels of the chemical in the brain higher.

Finding molecules that bind to the active site of a protein is difficult, and some processes cannot be blocked in the traditional way. In some cases, it would be more desirable to destroy the protein than disrupt it. That's where RNAi comes in. RNA is the single-stranded cousin of DNA. It is the molecule that directs the middle steps of protein production. By introducing the right bits of RNA into a cell, a protein could be destroyed. Since genes are chemical instructions calling for the cell to produce a protein, RNAi would essentially give physicians the power to turn off a gene. That would be an enormous tool for physicians.

Already, Swiss researchers have used RNAi to slow the progression of amytrophic lateral sclerosis, better known as Lou Gehrig's disease, in mice. The technique has also been used successfully in monkeys, turning off a gene that is critical to the metabolism of cholesterol. As a result, the monkeys' cholesterol levels were cut by two-thirds, according to the online version of the journal *Nature.* As I write this, human trials are underway for a pair of RNAi drugs to treat macular degeneration, the most common cause of blindness in adults. The drugs are designed to block production of proteins that trigger the disease. Needless to say, if the trials are successful, it would be a huge boost not only for those suffering from macular degeneration but for medicine in general. RNAi could be a powerful tool in modern medicine's arsenal of weapons to fight diseases and of course aging.

Because genes code for proteins, each longevity gene Barzilai finds may offer the chance for a pharmaceutical intervention to help ward off the ravages of time.

"Everything we've found so far can be a target of drug therapies," he says. Unfortunately, drug companies have not shown much interest. "The problem with aging is you don't show results the next day. It takes eight to ten years." Therefore, the cost to test a potential antiaging drug is around $500 million.

That isn't to say drug companies are not interested in coming up with drugs to help people live longer. One drug company is already producing a drug that raises HDL, and *Business Week* reports that Pfizer spent $800 million to develop a pill that combines an HDL-raising pill with its blockbuster drug atorvastatin (Lipitor), which lowers LDL cholesterol. Unfortunately, the trial failed.

Befriending Bacteria

Researchers are dreaming up other novel ways to keep us healthy in the twenty-first century. Bacteria are generally not considered our friends. After all, they are the cause of a host of illnesses, from food poisoning to strep throat. Researchers are developing ways to manipulate bacteria to use them as ways to fight cancer and tumors. Here's how. *Salmonella* is famous for its power to cause food poisoning and the misery that goes with it. The bacterium also thrives in human tumors. Human trials are under way with *Salmonella* that has been modified to destroy tumor cells. Investigators have started animal studies to determine whether the toxin-producing bacterium *Clostridium novyi* could be used to melt the dead interiors of tumors. And they are looking at altering *Listeria monocytogenes*, the cause of a deadly form of food poisoning, to make it appear more like tumor molecules as a way to trick the body's own defenses into attacking tumors.

Using the bacteria already living in our bodies to promote

our health has also attracted attention among researchers. Jeffrey Gordon, director for the Center for Genome Sciences at Washington University in St. Louis, thinks we might be able to use the bacteria in our guts to adjust our metabolism in a way that will keep us from gaining weight. Prebiotics and probiotics are very sterile sounding names for ways to manipulate our gut bacteria. The human gut is home to 10 trillion to 100 trillion microbes, from five hundred to one thousand species. Together, these bacteria, archaea (bacterialike creatures that live in extreme environments), and viruses outnumber our own cells by a factor of ten, but until recently, very little was known about them.

These species of bacteria—together known by the pleasant-sounding name microflora—are more than parasites, though. They break down otherwise indigestible plant fibers into nutrients we can use. For example, microbes in our bodies break down polysaccharide, a carbohydrate in foods ranging from breads to pasta. Microbes also help us store fat.

All of us do not have the same bacteria in our guts, though. We are microbe-free in the womb, but start acquiring bacteria from the moment we head down the birth canal. We wind up with a unique combination of microflora, though there is a constant flux in our microscopic squatters. If these bacteria are particularly good at breaking down food and storing it as fat, then we might be more prone to obesity. By one estimate, differences in the bacteria in people's digestive tracts may allow some people to eat 30 percent more calories daily than another without gaining weight.

What if we could manipulate the microbes? Could we

change the microflora in a way that would reduce the number of calories stored as fat? Would we be less prone to gaining weight? These are questions that have researchers excited, and they bring us back to probiotics and prebiotics.

Probiotics contain live bacteria and other microbes that are designed to be beneficial to our health. You may never have consciously consumed a probiotic, but you almost certainly have done just that. That's because yogurt contains the live bacterium *Lactobacillus acidophilus*. Probiotics live in other fermented dairy products as well. Yogurt has been touted for years as a food linked to long life, and *L. acidophilus* has been shown to enhance the body's immune response and raise levels of cytokines, messenger molecules that help regulate the activities of the immune system. Proponents of probiotics say we should be particularly concerned about having low levels of friendly bacteria in our guts after taking a course of antibiotics, if we have been eating poorly, or if we have been suffering from diarrhea.

Prebiotics are nonliving dietary supplements that selectively promote the growth of bacteria in your colon. You are essentially feeding the bacteria in your intestine the way you would feed a pet. Of course, we still don't know a whole lot about the creatures inside us. We do know microbial genes outnumber our own by a factor of one hundred. That's why Gordon likes to refer to these gut dwellers as "this vast community." He talks about them the way you or I might talk about a sprawling suburb you'd visited only once or twice. He also likes to talk about the human body as a "superorganism," because we are a combination of species (bacterial and human) sharing the same body.

Because they are so integral to the digestive process, Gordon thinks we might be able to enlist these microbes in our battle of the bulge. Gordon has been raising germ-free mice in a sterile lab. Without the benefit of gut bacteria helping them digest food, the germ-free mice are slim compared to genetically identical mice that are not kept in the sterile environment. In fact, these germ-free mice are able to gorge themselves and not get fat. When they are returned to a normal, germ-filled environment, however, they gain weight as readily as the other mice. Gordon thinks the role of the bacteria goes beyond digestion. He says gut bacteria also suppress a key gene in mice. The gene, which goes by the acronym *FIAF*, inhibits fat storage. Suppressing the *FIAF* (fasting-induced adipocyte factor protein) allows more fat to be stored. Germ-free mice do not suppress this protein, which means they are able to stay thin.

"We are at an amazing time for the understanding of self," Gordon says. "We're entering a phase of personalized nutrition."

Gordon says we might someday be able to manipulate "the microbial community or use microbes as teachers to see how they manipulate our biology, use them as a way to set up therapeutic targets." In other words, if we can't train them to digest our food in a way that doesn't promote fat storage, we might be able to learn from them to mimic what the more beneficial microbes are doing.

Converting Viruses

Viruses, too, may someday be enlisted as friends rather than foes. Researchers are investigating ways to use modified viruses as a potent delivery system to fight cancer. In 1997, British doctors received special permission from the United Kingdom's medical authorities to inject live herpes simplex virus in the brain of a twenty-one-year-old man with an aggressive form of brain cancer called a glioma. The treatment had never been tried anywhere in the world. It worked. The tumor went away, and the man who had been given four months to live was reportedly alive and well at this writing.

S. Moira Brown, who headed the University of Glasgow team that pioneered treatment with HSV1716, started a company to capitalize on the research, Crusade Laboratories. The U.K. company removes a protein from the herpes virus that causes it to grow. When it's injected, the virus steals this same protein from cancer cells, which ultimately causes the tumor to shrink and sometimes disappear. The goal is to kill the cancer cells. When the herpes virus reaches healthy cells, which do not have this growth driver, the virus stops spreading.

Crusade Laboratories has received approval in Europe to use the herpes simplex virus in treating gliomas. Crusader also has clinical trials under way in which they are using the virus in treating ovarian and other cancers. Researchers in the United States are also working on what are called virotherapies for brain and liver cancers.

Virotherapy holds promise because viruses are able to target cancer cells with pinpoint accuracy and cause few side effects. The ability to destroy cancer cells and leave healthy cells alone sets virotherapies apart from chemotherapy and radiation therapy, which are far less precise. By one estimate, chemotherapy agents kill about six cancer cells for every healthy cell killed. By comparison, viruses kill more than one thousand cancer cells for every healthy cell killed.

Replaceable You

Ray Kurzweil is among those who are thinking bigger. They believe we will someday be able to use our own cells to build replacement organs. When our heart or liver or kidneys or lungs become old, he and others believe we will someday be able to replace them. Dr. Anthony Atala at Wake Forest University in Winston-Salem, North Carolina, made history recently by growing a new bladder using a patient's own cells. By doing so, he became the first scientist to grow a human organ in a laboratory and transplant it into a human.

To investigate, we talked to one of his patients, a sixteen-year-old named Kaitlyne McNamara. She was born with spina bifida, a rare birth defect that stunts brain and spinal cord development. As she grew, McNamara's parents realized her bladder was not functioning properly. It turned out her bladder was about the size of a thimble and could not hold normal amounts of fluid. What didn't fit in her bladder flowed back toward her kidneys. Eventually, she would experience a bladder burst, resulting in embarrassing accidents she could not control. To make matters worse, her kidneys were becoming damaged. Doctors gave her the option of forming a new bladder out of a piece of intestine, a surgery with potential complications, or trying an experimental procedure and growing a new bladder using her own cells. She went with Atala, one of seven patients to try the new technique. All seven report their bladders hold more fluid, and they have fewer problems with incontinence.

Atala takes a small piece of the patient's bladder—less than the size of a postage stamp—and teases out muscle and bladder cells, which he grows in a petri dish. When there are enough cells, they are layered onto a three-dimensional mold shaped like a bladder and allowed to grow. Several weeks later, the cells have produced a bioengineered bladder, which is grafted onto the patients' own bladder. Atala is by no means alone in this field. Cartilage cells are being taken from patients, grown, and reimplanted. So are pieces of skin for burn victims. And this is just the beginning.

There is plenty of research still to be done before organs more complicated than the bladder are grown in the lab. Also, even with his remarkable feat in bioengineering, we need to remember that Atala did not replace the patient's entire bladder, which would require sophisticated surgery to attach the bladder to the ureters, the tubes that carry urine from the kidneys to the bladder. He took the new bladders and grafted them onto the existing ones.

The true holy grail is the creation of entirely new organs and tissue using the patients' own stem cells. These are the generic balls of cells smaller than a grain of rice that develop a few days after conception and are capable of becoming any of the two hundred or so kinds of cells in the body. Skin, bone, heart, lung, and brain all emerge from these versatile, virgin cells—essentially the body's master cells. Growing a new heart or kidney or liver from stem cells would result in a new organ free of any risk of rejection.

To do this, scientists would take a single cell from your arm or somewhere else on your body, remove the DNA-containing nucleus, and implant it in a donor egg cell that has had the nucleus removed. It would be grown for five to seven days, until the embryonic cells form. From there, the cells would be given specific nutrients and growth factors to create the desired type of cells. Creating an embryo simply for using its cells is something President Bush and others find morally objectionable, but scientists around the world are moving forward with the research. Given all the publicity and promise of stem cells, it's hard to believe human embryonic stem cells were only discovered in 1998.

An embryo is not the only place to harvest stem cells, though. They also come from bone marrow, the umbilical cord, and other tissues, but these alternatives appear to be more limited than embryonic stem cells in their ability to develop into different types of cells. Stem cells have been at the center of a great deal of hope and hype, clinical research, and controversy in recent years, but stem cell therapy is nothing new. It has been around and saving the lives of cancer patients for thirty years. It's called the bone marrow transplant, used in patients whose marrow tissue has been destroyed by chemotherapy or radiation therapy.

Stem cells' power to rejuvenate has come into sharp focus recently. There is hope stem cell treatments can be used for people suffering from the devastating and progressive Parkinson's disease. Others envision using stem cells to cure type 1 diabetes, which is caused by the loss of insulin-producing cells in the pancreas called islets. There is also the hope that stem cells could help people paralyzed by spinal cord injuries walk again. Already, researchers at the University of California, Irvine have reported that paralyzed rats treated with a stem cell therapy were able to walk. Stem cells have also shown promise in treating diabetic mice and helping rats and mice with conditions mimicking Alzheimer's and Parkinson's.

As I write this, Geron, a California biopharmaceutical company, claims to be close to filing for permission to conduct the first human trials on an embryonic stem cell therapy for spinal tissue repair. Other American researchers also say they are close to asking the FDA for permission to begin testing stem cell–based therapies for macular degeneration, heart muscle repair, and regenerating damaged skin. Others have "trained" embryonic stem cells to become most of the cell types affected by Parkinson's.

Other uses envisioned for stem cells include giving cystic fibrosis sufferers new lung tissue, the blind new cornea or retina tissue, the deaf new hair cells in the inner ear, the bald new hair follicles, type 2 diabetics new insulin-producing cells in the pancreas. The elderly could benefit from replacing diseased or worn-out brain cells, muscle, bone, cartilage, and skin. The possibilities are legion. There is even talk that stem cells could be used to grow new teeth.

Probably the boldest prediction of all is the potential for stem cells to create entirely new organs. If you suffer from heart disease, a new heart could be grown from your own cells. This would bring us closer to Ray Kurzweil's analogy of fixing problems in the body the way we are now able to fix problems in a house. It would solve the problem of one organ in your body aging faster than the rest of you. It squarely puts us in the realm of practical immortality.

Despite the enormous amount of media attention surrounding stem cell research, we are probably years away from any homegrown organs, or any of the other potential medical uses for stem cells for that matter. Still, early research offers a glimpse at the potential of stem cells. For example, embryonic stem cells can be made in a laboratory dish to grow into heart muscle cells that clump together and beat in unison. Taking that heart tissue and implanting it in a way that helps a patient with a diseased heart adds layers of complexity to the challenge, though.

Grow Your Own

There is another possible way to replace digits and limbs and maybe even portions of damaged organs that has been largely overlooked because of all the hoopla over stem cells—regrow our own. It can be done. Humans can regrow the liver even if most of it is removed in surgery. We can also regenerate blood and the outermost layer of skin. Children can even regrow the tip of a finger, from the base of the nail up. Of course, this is nothing compared with the salamander, which can regrow entire limbs. Amphibians like the salamander and certain fish can regrow other body parts, too, like the intestine or the spinal cord, even part of the heart. They do this by converting mature cells at the site of the injury to immature cells, which clump together into something called a blastema. The blastema, in turn, starts regrowing the missing body part.

Humans and other mammals scar at the site of a wound instead of converting mature cells to immature ones and regenerating tissue. Some scientists think we evolved this way because it reduces the chances of developing cancer and allows us to have a more robust immune system. But researchers are now studying the chemical processes that cause organs to grow in embryos. They think if they are able to develop a drug therapy that mimics the chemical signals orchestrating organ growth in embryos, then adults with kidney failure, for example, would be able to grow a new kidney. Tests of one such protein, named bone morphogenic protein-7, suggest it could potentially reverse tissue damage and scarring and improve function in patients with kidney disease.

The notion that mammals could potentially regrow organs received a boost in 2005, when a strain of lab mouse known as MRL showed the ability to grow back amputated digits and even portions of the heart, liver, and brain. Even more astonishing, injecting cells from the MRL mice into normal mice gave the previously unremarkable mice the power to regenerate tissue. So we are one step closer to achieving practical immortality and chasing life.

Slowing the Clock

Some investigators think we need to dig deeper to determine how to chase life by slowing the aging process. They think the root cause of aging lies in oxidative damage to the mitochondria, the cells' sausage-shaped power plants. Rejuvenating the mitochondria will turn back the hands of time, they reason. Here's why: Each mitochondrion has its own DNA, separate from the DNA in the nucleus of the cell. Because this small, circular strand of DNA is where energy is being produced in the cell, it is subject to point-blank exposure to free radicals and the mutations they cause. To make matters worse, mitochondria do not have the same elaborate mechanisms for repairing DNA damage as the cell's nucleus; they are copied more frequently than nuclear DNA, and they are replicated by an enzyme that is more error prone than its counterpart in the nucleus. It shouldn't be a surprise, then, that mutations accumulate quickly in mitochondrial DNA. The elderly generally have an array of mutations in their mitochondrial DNA. Scientists have even tested the same people fifteen years apart and shown the buildup of mitochondrial mutations. When mutations hit a critical level, energy production in the cells falls and finally, the cells self-destruct. When cells start dying off faster than they are replaced in the brain or heart or some other organ, the result is the loss of function that most of us think of as aging.

Researchers have started trying to manipulate the mitochondria. They've created mice more prone to developing mutations. As a result, these mice die young and develop many of the telltale signs of aging at a relatively early age, such as hair loss, stooped posture, hearing loss, and osteoporosis. That alone doesn't prove mitochondrial damage from free radicals causes aging. What researchers did next, though, certainly adds weight to their argument. Remember catalase (chapter 3), the enzyme that fights free radicals? When the gerontologist Peter Rabinovich and his team at the University of Washington got more catalase to the mitochondria, the mice lived 20 percent longer, and such age-related problems as heart disease developed later than normal. For now, delivering catalase to the mitochondria is incredibly difficult, and we are unlikely to be taking any sort of catalase treatment to boost our mitochondria anytime soon.

Cracking the Code

At each end of twenty-three pairs of chromosomes is a string of DNA that for years scientists assumed was genetic gibberish. These are called telomeres. Telomere sequences are repeated over and over, comprising ten thousand nucleotides. Telomeres cap the end of each chromosome, which contains our body's DNA. Each time the cells divide, the telomere sequence shortens. Telomere loss is steady over time. When they get short enough, the DNA cannot fold properly, and the cells stop dividing. This takes 290 or so days in the somatic cells in the body (the cells that are not involved in reproduction). All it takes is a single telomere on one chromosome becoming too short, and that's the end of cell division. Also, the distance from the gene to the end of the telomere appears to affect how the gene acts—and may play a role in aging.

The length of the telomeres on our chromosomes is linked to

longevity. On average, people with longer telomeres live longer than those with shorter telomeres. Not surprisingly, women lose telomeres at a slower rate than men. They also live longer. People with coronary artery disease, in general, have shorter telomeres. Women with chronically ill children have shorter telomeres than other women. Because we lose telomeres at a predictable rate, these women's cells were said to be nine to seventeen years older than that of other women under less stress. Having shorter telomeres also appears to increase the risk of infection.

Now researchers are measuring telomeres for signs how far our biological clocks have wound down. For example, Tim Spector of St. Thomas' Hospital in London measured the length of the telomeres at the end of chromosomes in the white blood cells of 1,122 women whose ages ranged from eighteen to seventy-six. Spector found the telomeres of the youngest women were about 7,500 base pairs long. Their length declined by an average of twenty-seven base pairs a year, but lifestyle could dramatically speed up the "clock." Spector used these measurements as his timetable for aging and concluded, for example, that smokers were biologically older than nonsmokers by 4.6 years on average, while the obese were 8.8 years older than those women who were lean. An obese smoker was, by Spector's reckoning, at least ten years older than a lean nonsmoker. One day, researchers hope that an enzyme, appropriately named telomerase, will allow them to reverse the process and cause the telomeres to maintain or grow in length. This could allow the creation of the perfect immortal cell and be the key to chasing life.

In the future, scientists will attempt to alter the cells' clocks by lengthening the telomeres to extend the life of the cells. The goal is to make an immortal cell, but we should be wary of freeing cells from their own natural life spans. We are all familiar with cells that are immortal. They are called cancer cells. The trick will be how to rejuvenate our cells selectively without unleashing "the beast." Because we have so many cells relative to most other species and because we live so long, we may need telomere shortening to counteract cancer.

Nanotechnology

As I mentioned, the final bridge in Ray Kurzweil's vision of future immortality is nanotechnology. This is the stuff science fiction is made of. He and others see atomic-scale engineering as a way to reprogram systems in our bodies. Microscopic nanobots will navigate through our bloodstreams, combating pathogens, correcting DNA mutations, and reversing the aging processes. They will also replace our digestive system and our heart, taking over the job of moving oxygen and carbon dioxide around our bodies. He even predicts nanobots will circulate in our brains, making us smarter. Kurzweil refers to this transformation as replacing version 1.0 of the human body with version 2.0.

Already, scientists have developed nanotechnologies that deliver insulin to diabetic rats via capsules with pores only 7 nanometers across, inject drugs to small tumors via microscopic spinning screws, and capture individual cells in microteeth. They have even crafted a micromachine that is part muscle tissue, part machine and is fueled by glucose. There are dozens of companies and research labs devoted to nanomedicine, and new breakthroughs emerge almost daily.

In one example of Kurzweil's predictions moving toward reality, researchers at the Massachusetts Institute of Technology have developed a technique that allows nanoparticles to group together inside tumors. The mass of nanoparticles is large enough to be detected by an MRI machine.

The Big Freeze

Of course, if you don't think any of this is going to work out, you can always try to call the biological equivalent of a time-out. Make arrangements to have your body frozen, with instructions to thaw you out when science has advanced enough to bring you back to life and keep you alive indefinitely.

For a news story, we talked to Brian Harris, a twenty-nine-year-old father who has made arrangements to have his body frozen when he dies. Harris told me he is looking forward to meeting his great, great, great, great, great-grandchildren. Harris is one of a small group of people, perhaps numbering one thousand, who call themselves cryonicists. As soon as they are legally dead, the freezing process begins. Ideally, the process would begin within minutes of death. The goal is to keep the tissue alive. With that in mind, the body's blood and much of its water are replaced to prevent tissue-destroying ice crystals from forming. When the freezing process is complete, the bodies—or sometimes just the head—are stored in liquid nitrogen in containers that resemble giant thermos bottles. This is not cheap. At Alcor Life Extension Foundation in Arizona, which may be the largest company catering to cryonicists, it costs $150,000 to store the whole body; $80,000 for the head and brain. More than seven hundred people have signed on with Alcor to be cryopreserved when they die. Among Alcor's seventy-three current clients is Ted Williams, the baseball great, who died in 2002. A similar company with the optimistic name Suspended Animation Inc. opened in Florida in 2005.

Surgeons are now exploring ways to place cooled patients into suspended animation—heart stopped, blood drained from the body, no electrical activity in the brain. Already, as neurosurgeons we are able to induce comas in patients and have even stopped their hearts and brains using a combination of medications and induced hypothermia. This is useful if the neurosurgeon is, for example, clipping a hard-to-reach brain aneurysm. There is no blood flowing through the brain, so there will be no bleeding as the surgeon performs the operation. The ability to stop all activity in the body is still a work in progress, currently being tested on pigs. If surgeons are able to slow all metabolic activity to a crawl for hours while they repair wounds and other injuries, what about taking it to the next level and suspending that life indefinitely—or until science catches up with whatever ails the patient?

Of course, technology is nowhere near ready to revive those who are dead and frozen. Most organs donated for transplant can only be preserved for twenty-four hours—less for hearts and more complex organs—and they are not frozen and revived. Still, hope—if not the cryonicists themselves—springs eternal.

"I think that reviving people that are cryopreserved is almost inevitable in some way or another, just like going to Mars is inevitable," Dr. Steve Harris, Alcor's medical director, told us. Some believers in cryonics have even made financial plans for the future by setting up "personal revival trusts," nest eggs for their reanimation.

Despite everything you have just read, I am not recommending you pull out your checkbook or start a cryonics savings account. While I do have faith in the future and the promise of science, I think we have a long way to go with simply realizing and harvesting our own potential. If you can do that, then your future is already here.

CHAPTER 10

Chasing Life

It is probably reasonable to assume that if you purchased this book, you are looking for ways to prolong your life and maybe even improve it. You may have a good reason to start thinking about this now. Maybe you woke up one day and found another gray hair or an extra wrinkle while staring in the bathroom mirror. Maybe you endured the tragic loss of someone close to you. Perhaps your situation is even more serious, and you are reading this book from your hospital bed or at home after a close call with your health. Every day, we have brushes with mortality, and they remind us how precious our lives really are. The truth is there are so many things I can't help you control. Life will deal you obstacles and challenges, which you will try to overcome the best you can.

This book, though, is about the things you can and should control. Taking a hard look at all the simple changes you can make in your life today makes me realize that we are already on the road to a practical immortality. We are already in the driver's seat when it comes to seriously controlling our own health. You have no idea what your body and your mind are capable of delivering for you. No, you don't have to wait for the promise of stem cells or cryonics, and I won't ask you to go out and buy hundreds of dollars worth of supplements. And we won't resign ourselves to the destiny of our genetics.

All over the world and right in your backyard, there are people who are steadily pushing back the frontier of aging. They are not content to simply wither away, becoming frail and feeling worthless. Instead, they are achieving a sort of practical immortality—living as long as they want to live and dying only when they are through living.

It does involve understanding what an athlete who never competed until the age of 86 can teach us about living gracefully through strenuous exercise. It may also involve getting to know an Okinawan who still works a steady job and has a new boyfriend, despite the fact that she is 103. It might even require spending a day with my friend Leonard Abraham, who at 95 still drives around in his sports car and loves climbing stairs every day as part of his exercise routine. They are all chasing life, and they are not even close to being done with their chase.

I decided to chase life for my new daughter, Sage. She has grown up a lot, even during the time she has watched me pounding away on the keyboard, writing this book. For her, every day, I have started to make smarter choices about the foods I eat and the number of calories I consume. I have thrown out some of those supplements I used to take and added more nutritional yet tasty food to my diet—at least seven different-colored foods each and every day. Admittedly, some of those foods and colors are red wine and brown chocolate. I try to surprise my body every day with new, challenging exercises, always including the all-important upper body training. I know it will help me ward off respiratory diseases later in life, and it has helped me find my old college physique again.

My attitude has somehow changed for the better as well. I don't become as easily fatigued or stressed at the end of the day. In part, it is because I know too much stress can shorten my life. It is also in part because I know as a result of following the advice in this book, my life will be longer, and I will have been successful in my chase for life. In this book, I have offered you the very best advice on what you can start doing today to chase life in a way that is simple and rises above the clutter of the plethora of advice out there. Everything you have just read is both important and factual and will in fact help improve and lengthen your life.

Immortality is on the horizon, and it is within our reach for the first time. The path to immortality will not always be easy, but for Sage and for me, it is worth it. I am sure you feel the same way. There is nothing more important.

RESOURCES

We live in an era when a wealth of knowledge beyond the dreams of scholars working only a generation ago is at our fingertips. The trick on the World Wide Web is not finding information, but locating information you can trust. Here are a few Web sites that offer solid information that can assist you as you chase life and try to live the longest, healthiest life possible.

The American Academy of Family Physicians
This comprehensive Web site bills itself as health information for the whole family, and it really does provide facts and advice on a range of health conditions and concerns, from childbirth through old age. There is also a "Smart Patient Guide" that contains advice on how to talk to your family doctor, ways to reduce your risk of falling victim to a medical error, and information about Medicare Part D, among other things.
www.familydoctor.org

American Cancer Society
The American Cancer Society has a Web site with a wealth of information about ways to reduce your risk of cancer and information about a myriad of cancers. The Web site also has information about the latest research and about how to get support if you have cancer.
www.cancer.org

American Diabetes Association

Given that as many as six million diabetics in the United States do not know they have the disease, it's important for Americans to get as much information on diabetes as possible. The American Diabetes Association has general information about the cause of diabetes and its symptoms. There is also a diabetes risk test on the site.
www.diabetes.org

American Heart Association

Learning the risks and signs of a heart attack or stroke may save your life. The American Heart Association's Web site has a well-written, concise list of symptoms for heart attack and stroke, as well as information about a number of other diseases and conditions. It also includes an A–Z encyclopedia, so you can look up Raynaud's syndrome, bacterial endocarditis, and hundreds of other terms.
www.americanheart.org

American Lung Association

Despite the warnings and all the early deaths every year in the United States and around the world caused by smoking, it's hard to believe people are still doing it. Quitting is extremely hard for many smokers. The American Lung Association site has links to information that can help smokers stop. There is also information about asthma, allergies, and lung cancer.
www.lungusa.org

The Centers for Disease Control and Prevention
The nation's health watchdog has the latest information about disease outbreaks and flu vaccines, but there is also plenty of other information on the CDC's Web site, including information about high blood pressure, breast cancer, bone health, physical activity, and nutrition.
www.cdc.gov

Food and Drug Administration
If you're looking for information about the side effects of or warnings about a specific prescription drug, the Center for Drug Evaluation and Research at the FDA has a database you can search. The site holds a wealth of other information, but it is often difficult to find.
www.fda.gov/cder/index.html

Harvard School of Public Health
This well-organized, well-written Web site, called "The Nutrition Source: Knowledge for Healthy Eating," answers frequently asked questions, such as, "What is the best way to lose weight?" and "Where do sugar-free products . . . fall in the Healthy Eating Pyramid?" There are separate sections containing information about protein, fiber, fruits and vegetables, calcium and milk, carbohydrates, alcohol, vitamins, and more.
www.hsph.harvard.edu/nutritionsource

Healthfinder

If you don't know where to start looking for information relating to your health, the federal Office of Disease Prevention and Health Promotion Web site is a good place to start. The site offers links to more than 1,800 agency and organization Web sites that have reliable health information on any disease, condition, or injury you can imagine. There is also an A–Z drug database on the site, which includes information on thousands of prescription and over-the-counter medications.
www.healthfinder.gov

HealthierUS

Put together by the Executive Office of the President and the U.S. Department of Health and Human Services, this site offers general information on how to live a more healthy life. It contains information about diet and fitness. The site also contains information about ways to promote healthy lifestyles in children and adolescents.
www.healthierus.gov

KidsHealth

This comprehensive site dedicated to children's health has information tailored for parents, children, and teens. The Web site, from the Nemours Foundation, also includes questions and answers for these groups. As an example of how the information is geared toward particular age groups, on the parents' section of the site, you'll find "Can I keep my cat now that I'm pregnant?" On the teen section, you'll find "Can I pierce my

own eyebrow?" For kids, there is a section on how to stay safe on the playground.
www.kidshealth.org

The Lance Armstrong Foundation
Started by the world's most famous cancer survivor, the Lance Armstrong Foundation has a wealth of information about cancer and the latest clinical trials. The foundation also underwrites a phone number (listed on the site) that connects cancer patients to educational assistance, qualified referrals, and counseling services.
www.livestrong.org

Linus Pauling Institute
The Linus Pauling Institute at Oregon State University has a very clearly written Web site that summarizes the latest research on the health benefits (or lack thereof) of specific vitamins, minerals, foods, and other nutrients. The site also tells you what foods to consume if you want to eat certain nutrients and what happens if you don't eat enough of them. If you're interested in delving deeper into nutrition, this site goes into the chemistry and science involved in what we eat.
lpi.oregonstate.edu/infocenter/index.html

Mayo Clinic
The Mayo Clinic's well-designed Web site provides information on an incredible array of topics. You can look up a disease or condition, check symptoms, and read a first aid guide. There

is a section on managing conditions and another on living well. There is also a section that offers tips tied to health news. For example, the site has advice on how to avoid food poisoning at home in the wake of recent *E. coli* contamination in spinach from California.
www.mayoclinic.com

MedlinePlus

This Web site, put together by the National Library of Medicine and the National Institutes of Health, is an online entrée into the world's largest medical library. You can look up more than four hundred diseases and conditions; find information about herbs, supplements, and pharmaceutical drugs; and explore other resources. There are also online tutorials on a wide range of topics.
www.medlineplus.gov

Memorial Sloan-Kettering Cancer Center

This world-renowned cancer hospital has information on its Web site about herbs, botanicals, and other products, from AE-941 (shark cartilage) to *Zingiber officinale* (ginger). The site tells you, among other things, the food sources for these substances, how they work in the body, possible adverse reactions, and whether the herbs or botanicals have known interactions with other drugs.
www.mskcc.org/mskcc/html/11570.cfm

National Cancer Institute

This government site is loaded with information about various cancers, treatments, prevention, screening, and testing. There is an A–Z list of cancers and a compendium of cancers organized by location in the body. The Web site also offers a drug dictionary so patients and others can learn about the medications used in cancer treatments.

www.cancer.gov

National Institutes of Health Office of Dietary Supplements

For many of us, the information we have about dietary supplements seems to rely heavily on word of mouth. We hear thirdhand that some supplement will offer some health benefit. How do we know if what we hear is true? The NIH Office of Dietary Supplements will help you separate the myth from the facts. Click on Health Information and then Full List of Dietary Supplement Fact Sheets. Click on any one of them to learn how much—if any—is recommended in your diet, what food contains the supplement in question, what claims are being made about it, and whether those claims have any validity. The site also has information on the special needs of the elderly and how to spot health fraud.

dietary-supplements.info.nih.gov/index.aspx

National Institute on Aging

This government site has tips for healthy aging and offers a wide range of free publications about topics from Alzheimer's disease, to hormones and menopause, to aging and your eyes.

The Web site also has a detailed fitness program for the elderly and information about clinical trials looking for participants.
www.nia.nih.gov

National Sleep Foundation
If you are one of the tens of millions of Americans who have trouble falling or staying asleep, you will find information about our natural sleep rhythms and how sleep varies between genders and as we age on the National Sleep Foundation's Web site. The site also has information about such sleep disorders as sleep apnea.
www.sleepfoundation.org

National Women's Health Information Center
This Web site answers common questions women have about their health. Among the topics on this government site are diabetes, prenatal care, cervical cancer, breast cancer, breastfeeding, body image, menopause and hormone therapy, pregnancy, quitting smoking, and violence against women.
www.4women.gov

U.S. Department of Agriculture
If you want to know exactly what is in the food you eat, you can use the Department of Agriculture's database of thirteen thousand foods commonly eaten in the United States. The site will give you a nutrient profile by familiar portion sizes. You can also adjust the portion size. Want to know what's in 1 cup of almonds or 6 ounces of lean beef? This site will tell you every-

thing, from the calories and fat to the saturated fatty acids and vitamins. The Web address below is more than a mouthful, but the information you'll access is incredibly detailed.
199.133.10.140/codesearchwebapp/(owzbor45z4cyyx45rjqkz555)/codesearch.aspx

READING LIST

Abramson, John. *Overdo$ed America: The Broken Promise of American Medicine*. New York: HarperCollins, 2004.

Austad, Stephen N. *Why We Age: What Science Is Discovering about the Body's Journey Through Life*. Hoboken: John Wiley and Sons Inc., 1997.

Benson, Herbert. *The Relaxation Response*. New York: HarperTorch, 1976.

Campbell, T. Colin. *The China Study: The Most Comprehensive Study of Nutrition Ever Conducted and the Startling Implications for Diet, Weight Loss and Long-Term Health*. Dallas: BenBella Books, 2006.

Dement, William C. *The Promise of Sleep: A Pioneer in Sleep Medicine Explores the Vital Connection Between Health, Happiness, and a Good Night's Sleep*. New York: Dell, 2000.

Gilbert, Daniel. *Stumbling on Happiness*. New York: Knopf, 2006.

Hagwood, Scott. *Memory Power: You Can Develop a Great Memory—America's Grand Master Shows You How*. New York: Free Press, 2006.

Kurzweil, Ray. *The Singularity Is Near: When Humans Transcend Biology*. New York: Viking Adult, 2005.

Kurzweil, Ray and Terry Grossman. *Fantastic Voyage: Live Long Enough to Live Forever*. New York: Rodale Press, 2004.

McGaugh, James L. *Memory and Emotion: The Making of Lasting Memories*. New York: Columbia University Press, 2003.

Olshansky, S. Jay and Bruce A. Carnes. *The Quest for Immortality: Science at the Frontiers of Aging*. New York: W. W. Norton & Company, 2001.

Rolls, Barbara. *The Volumetrics Eating Plan: Techniques and Recipes for Feeling Full on Fewer Calories*. New York: Morrow Cookbooks, 2005.

Rolls, Barbara and Robert A. Barnett. *The Volumetrics Weight-Control Plan*. New York: HarperCollins, 2000.

Sapolsky, Robert M. *Why Zebras Don't Get Ulcers*. New York: W. H. Freeman and Co., 1993.

Small, Gary. *The Memory Prescription: Dr. Gary Small's 14-Day Plan to Keep Your Brain and Body Young*. New York: Hyperion, 2004.

Willcox, Bradley J., D. Craig Willcox, and Makoto Suzuki. *The Okinawa Program: How the World's Longest-Lived People Achieve Everlasting Health—And How You Can Too*. New York: Three Rivers Press, 2001.

INDEX

abdominal fat, 151–52, 154, 160, 170, 176
Abraham, Leonard, 179–81, 200–201
Abrahams, Richard T., 79
Abramson, Dr. John, 166–67
Acomplia, 210
adenosine triphosphate (ATP), 51
aerobic exercise, *see* exercise, aerobic
African Americans
  diabetes and, 170
  hypertension in, 155
  vitamin D and, 32–33
aging
  debate over the root of, 207
  degenerative diseases and, *see specific diseases, e.g.* cancer; heart disease
  the future, 203–34
  individual rate of, 9
  lifestyle and, *see* diet; exercise; optimism; smoking; stress
  memory and, *see* memory
  in other species, 9
  physical peak, 10
  symptoms of, 8–9, 207
air pollution, 127
alcohol consumption, 107
  cancer and, 127
  red wine, 14, 70–71, 213–14
Alcor Life Extension Foundation, 233
Alzheimer, Alois, 101–102
Alzheimer's Association, 94, 109
Alzheimer's disease, 14–15, 62, 101–16, 193
  aging as risk factor for, 8, 94
  beta-amyloid plaque buildup and, 102, 109, 112
  diet and, 106–109
  drugs for, 104
  education and work complexity and, 110–11, 113–16
  exercise and, 110
  genetics and, 103
  life circumstances and, 111
  oligomers and, 102–103
  stem cell research and, 14
  vaccine for, 105
American Cancer Society, 53, 127, 128, 132, 133, 136, 141–42, 144, 145, 239
American College of Cardiology, 163
American Diabetes Association, 169, 240
American Dietetic Association (ADA), 45
American Heart Association, 53, 155, 162, 240
American Plastics Council, 138
Andel, Ross, 111
anemia, 36–37
angiograms, 157
anterograde amnesia, 26–27
antidepressants, 196–97
anti-inflammatory agents, 108
antioxidants, 31–32, 45, 49–56, 69–70, 147
antiperspirants and cancer risk, 141
appetite
  drugs to moderate, 210
  memory and, 26–27
apple-shaped bodies, 152
Archives of Internal Medicine, 110, 185
aristolochic acid, 58
arrhythmias, cardiac, 156
artificial sweeteners, 108, 134–35, 175
Ashkenazi Jews, 211

INDEX

ashwaganda, 56
aspartame, 134
aspirin, 167–68
Atala, Dr. Anthony, 222–23
atherosclerosis, 156
atorvastatin (Lipitor), 166, 217
attitude, 13, 179–90, 194

Bacon, Roger, 69
bacteria, 217–20
Baltimore Longitudinal Study of Aging, 41
barbecuing meats, 133
Barzilai, Dr. Nir, 211–17
Benson, Dr. Herbert, 190–91, 194–95, 199
beta-carotene, 53, 107
bisphenol-A (BPA), 138–39
bladder cancer, 134
blood pressure, 71, 109, 162
  calorie restriction and, 40
  diet and, 35
  exercise and, 85
  hypertension, 112, 155–56, 157, 168, 169, 176, 212
blood sugar, 85, 173, 176
Blumberg, Jeffrey, 53–54, 62–63
body mass index (BMI), 170
body parts, replacement of, 222–27
Body Worlds: The Anatomical Exhibition of Real Human Bodies, 152–54
bone density scan, 65
bone marrow transplant, 224
bone mineral density, 35, 64–65, 83
bone morphogenic protein-7, 227
bovine growth hormone (BGH), 130–32
breakfast, 28
breast cancer, 17, 61, 84, 120, 126, 139, 142, 143, 146
Brigham and Women's Hospital, 159
Brigham Young University, 115
Brown, Laura, 47–48, 72
Brown, S. Moira, 221
Brown-Séquard, Charles Édouard, 68
Bryntsalov, Vladimir, 4
BusinessWeek, 217
Buzan, Tony, 99

calcium, 29, 32, 36, 64–65
Calment, Jeanne, 8, 14, 204
calorie restriction, 12–13, 20, 40–44, 209
  research on, 40–43
  side effects of, 43
calories in American diet, 21–22
Campbell, T. Colin, 141
cancer, 17, 52, 67, 205, 217
  aging as risk factor for, 8, 147–48
  controllable risk factors, 127–30
  delayed detection, 146–47
  diet and, 141–42
  early detection of, 127, 143–46
  exercise and, 142–43
  myths and facts, 130–41
  new treatments for, 126
  progress in war on, 119, 120
  soy products and, 61
  statistics, 119–20
  targeted molecular therapies for, 126
  virotherapies, 220–22
  see also specific types of cancer
Cancerel, 134
carbohydrates, 172–73
  processed foods and, 34
  unrefined, 20, 34, 173
catalase, 52, 55, 229
cell phones, cancer and, 135–37
centenarians, 211–14
Center for Science in the Public Interest, 162
Centers for Disease Control and Prevention, 88, 241
cervical cancer screening, 127, 143, 144
cervical cancer vaccine, 144
chemotherapy, 126, 221–22
chocolate, dark, 13, 69–70
cholesterol, serum, 71, 109, 156, 157, 163, 213–14
  "bad," *see* LDL cholesterol
  exercise and, 85

"good," *see* HDL cholesterol
statins to lower, 159, 165–67
cigarette smoking, *see* smoking
Citrus aurantium, 58
Cleveland Clinic Heart Center, 159
Clinton, Bill, 157
clopidogrel bisulphate (Plavix), 167, 168
clostridium novyi, 217
coffee, 14, 71
cognitive reserve, theory of, 114–15
colorectal cancer, 33, 71, 84, 120, 126, 133, 142, 143, 144
copper, diet high in, 109
cortisol, 186
C-reactive protein (CRP), 158–59
Crusade Laboratories, 221
cryonicists, 232–34
curcumin, 108
cyclamates, 134
cystic fibrosis, 225

dementia, 94
see also Alzheimer's disease; memory
dental checkups, 145
deodorants and cancer risk, 141
depression, 60, 109, 185, 186
placebo effect and, 196–97, 198–99
DHA (docosahexaenoic acid), 107
DHEA (dehydroepiandrosterone), 67–68
diabetes, 112, 169–77, 193, 205, 212
aging as risk factor for, 8
complications of, 168–69
diet and, 171–76
exercise and, 84
fiber and, 33
gestational, 169
prediabetes, 170
signs of, 169
statistics, 169
type 1, 224–25
type 2, 71, 112, 154–55, 169–77, 225
Diener, Ed, 188–89
diet
calorie restriction, *see* calorie restriction
cancer and, 141–42
degenerative diseases and, *see individual diseases*
diabetes and, 171–76
eating less, 12–13
energy dense foods, 24
heart disease and, 162–65
memory and, 106–109
minerals, *see individual minerals*
Okinawan, 20, 44–45
stop eating before your full, 24–28, 45
vitamins and, *see individual vitamins*
water content, foods with high, 24–25
see also specific foods and food groups
dioxins, 137–38
double blind study, 196
drug interactions, 57
Duke University Medical Center, 154

echinacea, 59
education, 187
Alzheimer's disease and, 110, 113–16
electron beam computed tomography (EBCT), 158
endometrial cancer, 145
Environmental Protection Agency, 139, 140
ephedra, 57, 58
epicatechin, 70
epinephrine (adrenaline), 192
Equal (sweetener), 134
esophagus, cancer of the, 120, 128, 142
European Institute of Cancer Research, 136
European Union, regulators in
aspartame and, 134
bovine growth hormone and, 131–32
genetically modified crops and, 132
exercise, 13, 22, 75–92, 186
abdominal fat and, 154, 160
aerobic, 81–82, 84, 88, 110
breathing, 84
daily activities as, 86, 89–90
expectations and goals, 86–87

INDEX

exercise (*cont.*)
  flexibility and, 83
  frequency of, 84
  at home, 83–84
  listening to your body, 88
  memory and, 106, 110
  mental, 100–101, 112–17
  motivating yourself, 85
  Okinawans and, 19–20, 110
  starting out, 83, 86
  strength training, 81, 82–84, 110, 160
  warming up, 84
  see also specific conditions affected by exercise, e.g. cancer; heart disease
Experimental Biology and Medicine, 58

Fantastic Voyage (Kurzweil), 204
fast foods, 23–24, 162
  choices among, 37–38
fasting, intermittent, 43
fat, body, 22
fats and oils, 22, 162
  hydrogenated, 162
  saturated, 108, 109
  sensory pleasure of, 38–39
  trans-fatty acids, 108, 109
FIAF (fasting-induced adipocyte factor protein), 220
fiber, dietary, 29, 33–34, 44, 163, 164
fight-or-flight response, 192–93
fish, 106–107, 163
  omega-3 fats in, 44
fish oil supplements, 62
flavonoids, 45, 70
fluoride and cancer risk, 141
folic acid, 37, 64, 112, 164
food additives and cancer risk, 141
Food and Drug Administration, 57, 104, 130, 131, 135, 138, 140, 141, 144, 210, 225, 241
Free Radical Biology and Medicine, 55
free radicals, 31–32, 43, 49–56, 207, 229
Fridovich, Irwin, 49, 50
fruits and vegetables, 24, 44–45, 127, 133
  antioxidants in, 45, 54
  cancer and, 142
  heart disease and, 162, 163–64, 165
  memory and, 107
  minerals in, 34, 35
  in Okinawan diet, 20
  processing's effects on nutritional value of, 29–30
  USDA recommended daily servings of, 45
Fuller, Ida May, 11
future of aging and longevity, 203–34

Gallup International, 190
garlic, 60
genetically modified organisms (GMOs), 132
genetics
  Alzheimer's disease and, 103
  heart disease and, 156, 157
  longevity and, 14, 208–209, 210–11
gestational diabetes, 169
ghrelin, 161, 210
Gingko biloba, 61, 109
ginseng, 60–61
glioblastoma, 121–25
gliomas, 221
glucosamine and chondroitin, 61–62
glutathione peroxidase, 52
glycemic index, 173–74
Gordon, Jeffrey, 218, 219–20
green tea, 14, 71
grilling meats, 133

Hagwood, Scott, 98–101, 116
Hammond, James, 75–78, 80, 90
happiness, *see* optimism
hara hachi bu, 20–28, 39, 45
Harris, Brian, 232
Harris, Dr. Steve, 234
Harvard School of Public Health, 32, 127, 241
Hassenbusch, Dr. Samuel, III, 121–25
HDL cholesterol, 40, 169, 213–14, 217

health span, 12
heart disease, 17, 67, 154, 155–68, 176, 205, 212
  aging as risk factor for, 8
  aspirin and, 167–68
  diet and, 32, 33, 62, 106, 162–65
  exercise and, 84, 160
  family history and, 156, 157
  homocysteine and, 112, 164
  optimism and, 184–85
  sleep and, 160–61
  smoking and, 161
  statins for, 159, 165–67
herbs and supplements, *see* supplements and herbs
heredity, *see* genetics
herpes simplex virus, 221
heterocyclic amines, 133
Hispanics, diabetes and, 170
HIV/AIDS, 205
hobbies, 13
homocysteine, 112, 164
Honolulu Heart Program, 165
hormesis hypothesis, 44
hormone supplements, 66–69
human growth hormone (HGH), 66–67, 68–69
human papillomavirus (HPV), 127
hypertension, 112, 155–56, 157, 168, 169, 176, 212

immortality
  history of quest for, 7–8
  practical, 12
immune system, 186
infant mortality rate, 10
infertility, 193
insulin, 169, 172, 173
International Health, Racquet & Sportsclub Association, 78
iron, 36–37

Jennings, Peter, 146
Joslin Guide to Diabetes, 174
Journal of Biological Chemistry, 50
Journal of Personality and Social Psychology, 183
Journal of the American College of Cardiology, 81, 158
Journal of the American Medical Association, 160

Kesler, Shelli R., 115
kidney cancer, 120
kidney disease, 176
King, Laura, 188–89
Kurzweil, Ray, 14, 174, 203–206, 222, 225–26

Lactobacillus acidophilus, 219
La Lanne, Jack, 8
Lancet, The, 127
LDL cholesterol, 61, 67, 158, 163, 213
  calorie restriction and, 40
  statins to lower, 159, 165–67
life expectancy
  active, 12
  changes in average, 10–11
  future of, 204
  in other developed countries, 14
life span, 8, 14, 204
Lind, James, 30
Linus Pauling Institute, 72, 243
Listeria monocytogenes, 217
liver cancers, 221
longevity
  genetics and, 14, 208–209, 210–11
  HDL and LDL cholesterol and, 213–14
  of Okinawans, 17–21
  research on peoples with extreme, 7–8, 211–14
lung cancer, 120, 128, 142, 146–47
lycopene, 29, 163
Lyubomirsky, Sonja, 188–89

McCabe, Micki, 146–47
McCord, Joe, 49, 50, 51, 52, 54–55, 71

INDEX

McGaugh, James, 96
McNamara, Kaitlyne, 222
macular degeneration, 31, 216, 225
magnesium, 29, 35
mammography, 143, 146
marriage
  happiness and, 187, 188
  risk of Alzheimer's disease and, 111
Massachusetts Institute of Technology, 232
Mayo Clinc, 72, 243–44
meats
  cooking at very high temperatures, 133
  nitrites in processed, 132–33
Mediterranean diet, 60, 106
memory
  Alzheimer's disease, *see* Alzheimer's disease
  appetite and, 26–27
  Baker/baker experiment, 96–97
  the brain as filter, 97–98
  emotional memories, 100
  exercise and, 110
  exercising your brain, 100–101, 112–17
  explanation of how it works, 95–96, 98
  supplements to improve, 61
  tricks, 99–100, 101
Memory Fitness Institute, 112–13
Memory Power (Hagwood), 99
microflora, 218–19
microwave cooking, cancer risk and, 137, 139, 140
Mind Body Medical Institute, 190, 199
minerals
  supplements, 62, 63–65
  see also individual minerals
mitochondria, 51–52, 88, 207, 228–29
Monsanto, 130, 131
Mortimer, James, 111
Moseley, Dr. Bruce, 197
multivitamins, 62, 63, 147

nanotechnology, 206, 231–32
National Cancer Act, 119
National Cancer Institute, 120, 134, 141, 245
National Center for Complementary and Alternative Medicine, 59, 61
National Health and Nutrition Examination Surveys, 23, 164–65
National Institute on Aging, 37, 40, 94, 182, 245–46
National Institutes of Health, Office of Dietary Supplements, 65, 72, 245
National Obesity Forum, 151–52
National Osteoporosis Foundation, 65
National Toxicology Program, 135
Nature, 70, 216
neuroplasticity, 115–16, 181–82
New England Centenarian Study, 213, 214
New England Journal of Medicine, 59, 65, 66, 158, 168
Nissen, Dr. Steve, 165–66
nitrites, 132–33
Nixon, Richard, war on cancer, 119, 120, 149
nocebo effect, 199
Northwestern University, 102–103
NutraSweet, 134
nutrition, *see* diet
Nutrition Today, 24

obesity and overweight, 22–23, 81, 109, 127, 133, 142–43, 168–69, 170, 176
  waist size, 151–52, 154
Okinawans, 17–21, 25, 27–28, 44–45, 110
Okushima, Ushi, 17–19
olfactory nerves, 39
oligomers, 102–103
omega-3 fatty acids, 44, 62, 107, 163, 165
  supplements, 73, 107
optimism, 13, 179–90
organic foods, 132
organs, replacement of, 222–27
osteoarthritis, 14–15, 82
osteoporosis, 36, 64–65, 83, 84
Overdo$ed America (Abramson), 166
overweight, *see* obesity and overweight
oxidative stress, 50, 228
Ozug, Chuck, 93–94

Page, Satchel, 181
Pap tests, 127, 144
Parkinson's disease, 8, 71
  diet and, 32
  stem cell research and, 14, 224, 225
PCBs in fish, 107
pear-shaped bodies, 152
perfluorooctanoic acid (PFOA), 140
personalized medicine, 206
pessimism, 185
  see also optimism
Pew Research Center, 187
Pfizer, 217
phthalates, 138
physical activity, *see* exercise
physical exam, annual, 145
Pittsburgh School of Public Health, 81
placebo effect, 60, 196–200
plastics, cancer risk of, 137–39
Plavix, 167, 168
pneumonia, 10, 82
polycyclic aromatic hydrocarbons, 133
Ponce de León, Juan, 7
portion sizes, 23–24, 25, 171
potassium, 29, 34, 165
Pozdnyakova, Tatyana, 79–80
prebiotics, 218–19
premenstrual syndrome (PMS), 193
probiotics, 218–19
processed foods, 34, 173
  meats, 133–34
prostate cancer, 17, 61, 120, 139, 144–45
Psychological Bulletin, 189
Psychological Science, 27

quality of life, 10

Rabinovich, Peter, 229
raloxifene (Evista), 104–105
Ravussin, Eric, 42
Redelmeier, Donald, 189
red wine, 14, 70–71, 213–14
Reeve, Dana, 146
relaxation response, 191, 194–95
Relaxation Response, The (Benson), 190–91
religion, 187
resources, 239–47
resveratrol, 70–71, 209–10
rimonabant, 210
rituximab (Rituxan), 126
RNA interference (RNAi), 215–16
Rolls, Dr. Barbara, 23–25
Rosin, Paul, 27
Running USA, 78–79
Rush University Medical Center, 113–14

saccharin, 134–35
Saint-John's-wort, 60
Salmonella, 217
SARS (severe acute respiratory syndrome), 205
scurvy, 30–31
Sequarine, 68
Seventh-Day Adventists, 171
sex, unsafe, 127
Singularity Is Near, The (Kurzweil), 204
SIR2 gene, 208–209
SIRT1 gene, 209
skin melanoma, 120, 145–46
sleep, 13
  appetite, and weight control, 160–61
  exercise and, 85
  stress and, 195–96
Small, Dr. Gary, 106, 112–13
smell, sense of, 38–39
smoking, 14, 52, 186, 230
  cancer and, 127, 128–30
  cessation treatments, 129
  dementia and, 108, 109
  heart disease and, 161
  secondhand smoke, 130
snacking, 28
social ties, 13, 20
soy products, 61
Spector, Tim, 230
spinal cord injuries, 225

INDEX

Stanford University, 115
statins, cholesterol-lowering, 159, 165–67
  for Alzheimer's disease, 104–105
Stein, Dr. Richard, 157
stem cells, 2–7, 14, 224–26
stomach cancer, 142
strength training, 81, 82–84, 110, 160
stress, 190–96
  defining, 191
  exercise to relieve, 85, 194
  fight-or-flight response, 192–93
  reduction techniques, 106, 191, 193–95
  sleep and, 195–96
stroke, 8, 17, 35, 67, 112, 154, 165, 167, 168, 184–85, 212
sun exposure, 52, 145–46
superoxidase dismutase (SOD), 49, 52, 55
supplements and herbs, 13, 47–74
  antioxidants, 49–56
  educating yourself, 72
  to fill voids in your diet, 63
  hormone replacement, 66–69
  popular, efficacy of, 59–62
  safety issues, 56–59
  vitamin and mineral, 62, 63–65
Sweet'N Low, 134–35

Taming the Beast, 121
taste, sense of, 38–39
Teflon, 139
telomeres, 148–49, 229–31
Tepliashin, Dr. Alexander, 2–7
testicular cancer, 120
testosterone, 66, 67
theory of cognitive reserve, 114–15
thyroid cancer, 120
thyroid hormones, 67–68
trans-fatty acids, 108, 109
triglycerides, 61
Tufts University, 82
turmeric, 14, 107–108
type 2 diabetes, 71, 112, 154–55, 169–77

U.S. Department of Agriculture, 21–22, 45, 246–47
U.S. Department of Health and Human Services, 186
University of California
  Davis, 71
  Irvine, 225
University of Kansas, 198
University of Toronto, portfolio diet, 165
USA Triathlon, 79

vegetables, *see* fruits and vegetables
virotherapies, 220–22
vitamin A, 29, 31, 52, 53
vitamin B_6, 64, 112
vitamin B_{12}, 37, 64, 112
vitamin C, 29–31, 52, 53, 107
vitamin D, 32–33, 64, 65
vitamin E, 29, 31–32, 52, 53, 107
vitamin supplements, 62, 63–65
Volumetrics Weight-Control Plan, The (Rolls), 24–25
von Hagens, Dr. Gunther, 152

waist size, 151–52, 154, 170, 176
Washington University, St. Louis, 40
water
  body functions requiring, 38
  foods with high-water content, 24–25
weight loss, 170–71
  calorie restriction and, 41
weight training, *see* strength training
Williams, Ted, 233
wine, red, 14, 70–71, 213–14
World Health Organization, 136
Wray, Dr. Nelda, 197

Yushchenko, Viktor, 4–5

ABOUT THE AUTHOR

SANJAY GUPTA, MD, is a practicing neurosurgeon and associate chief of neurosurgery at Grady Memorial Hospital and an assistant professor at Emory University Hospital in Atlanta. He is a columnist for *Time* magazine, a contributor to CBS News, and a chief medical correspondent at CNN, where he plays an integral role in the network's medical coverage, including daily reports, the half-hour weekend show *House Call with Dr. Sanjay Gupta*, and coverage of breaking medical news. He also cohosts *Accent Health* for Turner Private Networks, provides medical segments for the syndicated version of *ER* on TNT, and contributes health news stories to CNN.com. He recently launched a weekly podcast on iTunes called *Paging Dr. Gupta.*

Before joining CNN, Gupta was a neurosurgeon at the University of Tennessee's Semmes-Murphey clinic, and before that at the University of Michigan Medical Center. He became a partner in the Great Lakes Brain and Spine Institute in 2000, and in 1997, he was chosen as a White House Fellow, one of only fifteen fellows appointed. He served as special advisor to First Lady Hillary Rodham Clinton.

Gupta has been published in a variety of scientific journals and has received numerous accolades. In 2006, he won an Emmy Award and four National Headliner Awards, the most an individual journalist has ever received. In 2004, the Atlanta

Press Club named him Journalist of the Year. His coverage has led to prestigious Peabody and duPont awards for CNN. He has won the Humanitarian Award from the National Press Photographers Association, a Gold Award from the National Health Care Communicators, and a finalist honor for the International Health and Medical Media award known as the FREDDIE.

He is a member of several organizations, including the American Association of Neurological Surgeons, the Congress of Neurological Surgeons, and the Council of Foreign Relations. He is also a board member of Live Strong. Dr. Gupta is a certified medical investigator and a board-certified neurosurgeon. He is a diplomate of the American Board of Neurosurgery.